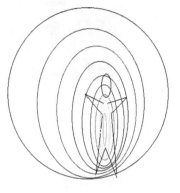

Total Wellness
Publishing

Where We Go From Here

Your Body's Best Kept Secrets Revealed

"Homeopathy has helped me transcend my life-long barrier of self-consciousness. I no longer worry about the expression of my thoughts, and people's reaction to them."

Mathew Engleman (Student)

"I have suffered from migraine headaches for years that were beginning to control my life. I tried cleansing, acupuncture, nutrition, deep tissue message therapy, reflexology, chiropractic adjustment and nothing helped. My next step was drug therapy, which I was trying to avoid because I was afraid that my concentration would be affected. The very first remedy I took got rid of my migraine in less than five minutes. I have been headache free since. I am extremely thankful to Michele Iqbal and homeopathy."

Linda Ann Carty
Doctor of Chiropractor

"Homeopathy has helped me in many ways. Mentally, I feel more self-confident and I know I think much more clearly. Physically, I have completely cleared a life-long problem with fluid retention and my menopausal symptoms, including the horrible hot flashes, are much much better. I'm feeling pretty good.

Shirley Garofalo, Hypnotherapist

"Recently, I severely burned my hand. Pain and blisters erupted immediately. I ran for the Cantharis 30X and took 2 pellets every 10 minutes for 1 hour. Within 2 hours the pain was minimal and by the next morning (8 hours later) there was no pain and there were no blisters. My example of the miracle of Homeopathy is rather dramatic, but serves to prove to me the reality of treating symptoms and taking charge of my continuing wellness.

Shelly B., Highland, California

"I was suffering from a series of nervous breakdowns and intense agitated depression when I first came to Michele. Within 45 minutes of taking my first remedy, the agitated depression abated and I was able to function again. I had tried homeopathy before so I was open to it, but with Michele, I had a sense I would be able to get rid of my problem. I continued to work with her for several months, and today I have no twinge of a problem. I have not had an episode in 2 years, it is completely reversed and I no longer live in fear. My problem was inherited, several people in my family have similar problems, and I am the only one who is free of symptoms without medication. I believe people should give it a try. It is not a quick fix, but over many months of working through symptoms, it does work."

Jeff Barone, Teacher

"I could write a tribute to homeopathy that would take up this entire book--I have so much to say about how it's helped me, my family, and my friends.

Over the years homeopathy has cured (yes, I do mean literally "cured") most of the many physical and mental ailments in my family. A short list includes: arthritis, depression, headaches, allergies, anxiety attacks, bipolar mood swings, and even lowly canker sores. This list doesn't include the many, many acute health problems that have been quickly taken care of, or the minor, chronic problems that you get so used to you don't even notice until they're gone.

I can literally say that homeopathy has changed my life and the life of everyone in my family--and even a few friends. I don't think that's an exaggeration. Before homeopathy we had poor health and no real prospect of getting better. Since being treated with homeopathy, and now learning its use myself, we enjoy good physical and emotional health. None of us takes any medications. This is especially remarkable in my son's case, because every psychiatrist and neurologist you ask will tell you that there is no cure for bipolar disorder, obsessive/compulsive disorder, and all those things he was diagnosed with. They will tell you that the patient must be on medication for the rest of his life. Homeopathy works. No kidding."

Kim Foreman, Riverside, California

The Dr. Iqbal Book of Homeopathy
Part One:

Your Body's Best Kept Secrets Revealed

By Dr. Iqbal

Total Wellness Publishing
Fontana, CA

Dedicated to my husband
Muzaffar Iqbal
who has always supported my
homeopathic studies.

Table of Contents

• Disclosure (please read)

Michele Iqbal is not a medical doctor and is not licensed as a medical professional in the State of California since no licensing is offered for homeopathy, but rather holds a Ph.D. from the National College of Homeopathy, Rawalpindi, Pakistan, a D.H.M.S (Diploma of Homeopathic Medical Sciences). This degrees allows for the use of the prefix "Dr".

Homeopathy is a branch of alternative healing using dietary supplements in which energy is used to assist the energy systems of the body with the process of healing. To accomplish this, homeopathy relies on the use of remedies that have been reduced from a material substance to their energy form by a process known as potentizing. Unlike other forms of medicine which rely on chemicals and physical manipulation of the body, homeopathy can not cause a condition that does not already exist.

The information in this book is for educational purposes only and is not to be construed as medical advice, nor should it be interpreted or used as a substitute for a qualified physician's evaluation or treatment. Those who purchase or download this book are urged to check their local and state regulations regarding any and all legalities concerning use of this information. Any information or concept taken from this book and used by any individual is done so at their own risk. Total Wellness Publishing and Michele Iqbal cannot be held legally responsible for the use, misuse or misinterpretation of remedy use.

This book is designed to provide information. It is not the purpose of this book to provide all the information available on the subject of homeopathy, but rather to complement and supplement other texts. Homeopathy is practiced from many different points of view and perspectives. Information in conflict with other explanations of homeopathy simply represents an additional point of view, which the reader is encouraged to evaluate.

Every effort has been made to make this book as complete and accurate as possible. However, mistakes can and do occur, both typographical and in content. The information contained in this book is accurate, to the best of our knowledge, as of the date printed.

The opinions express in the book are those of Michele Iqbal gained through many years of contemplation, experimentation and practice with homeopathy and do not reflect scientific thought or method.

Foreword

Let me make one thing perfectly clear. I do not do what you may think homeopathic practitioners do.

I do not want to see you in my practice. I don't have a practice.

I do not want you to tell me about your medical complaints. If you have complaints, see a doctor. If you have only a few annoyances you don't know what to do about, you are the one I want to talk to. Prevention is everything when it comes to long term good health and most people do not recognize the signs that indicate future problems.

I do not want you to replace your regular medicines with homeopathic remedies or dietary supplements. That is not possible and to think that it is creates a complete misunderstanding of what homeopathy can do.

I want you to realize that just because you do not feel sick, just because you have nothing concrete to complain about, just because you don't think about what may be in store for you in the future doesn't mean you should ignore the simple things I can teach you to stay healthy.

I hate anti-bacterial soaps and disinfectants. I don't believe in killing everything before it gets to you. In fact, this practice is very dangerous. Using anti-bacterial products creates super bugs. You need to allow your immune system to shake hands with germs and form defenses against them. Remember that old saying, "know thine enemy".

You won't catch me downing massive doses of Vitamin C, taking anti-oxidants or worrying about whether I eat fast food or not. I'm not a vegetarian. A completely vegetarian life style can make a person weak and vulnerable to injury and illness.

And you will never ever catch me in a room where an ozone producing air cleaning machine is running. I feel sick the minute I walk into such a place. These machines put a negative charge on air particles. Negative charged air particles neutralize the positive charge of the energy structures that control the human body. Spending time in a room filled with predominantly negative charged ozone eats away energy bodies causing the loss of mental functions and creating weaknesses that compromise immunity to serious illness. If you have one, turn it off—except maybe for short periods on days when the wind is blowing and allergens are more than usual.

Homeopathy is a tool to be used to restore the communication systems that run the human body. However, this book is not so much about homeopathy as it is about the way the body works, the way energy animates the material substance of the body and the way the mind gathers and uses information.

Attitudes toward information gathered through so called "psychic" means are changing. Most people no longer question whether psychic phenomenon exists and because of this we are seeing the development of a new era. The veil covering information that has been hidden from us and manipulated by authority figures is lifting. As we see glimpses of this long hidden more accurate data that is now flooding our media, we are losing tolerance for inaccuracies and the double talk of rhetoric. It is now clear that psychically accessed information can be used as a benefit. If all police departments used psychics and mediums to obtain information about crimes, maybe criminals would think twice before committing their acts. If doctors accepted that the human body is controlled by energy structures, new and more effective forms of treatment can be merged into conventional methods for the benefit of all.

The ancient Greeks attributed healing to the gods. Patients were expected to be asleep at the time a priest with a connection to the god who was to perform the healing came to visit. In the great healing Temples of Asclepios, any attempts to heal illness or change symptoms other than by the methods used in the priest/god manner were rejected as unconventional and contrary to accepted methods.

After the influence of the temples had dissipated and the methods and philosophies of the Hippocratic schools had gained acceptance, the art of healing by manipulating the body or using substances to change symptoms advanced to remarkable levels. However, the Black Plague epidemics of the dark ages killed the majority of the practicing physicians. This catastrophic event resulted in the loss of wisdom about the body and many effective healing methods. False assumptions about many procedures used prior to the loss of the properly trained doctors caused medicine to fall into a period where painful and often harmful procedures became common.

The Renaissance era brought back the scientific

method and advanced the medical sciences to a new level through the disciplines of investigation and experimentation. Most advances in modern medicine have been made by the methods developed at this time.

Since the beginning of the Christian era, there has been a separation between what the faith systems have stated about the nature of the soul and the medical system's assumption that human beings are composed of mostly material substance. The energetic nature of a human being, which is the result of the blending of the spirit that is the soul and the material body of flesh and blood, has never been fully appreciated. The ancients considered only the soul, modern medicine considers only the body. The understanding that human beings are a blend of body and soul is essential in maintaining good health.

The "New Age Movement" of the 1990's touched on the importance of the Soul/Body connection. However, most of the products and services offered were promoted out of context from their original use in the indiginous cultures of their origin and tauted in potencies or for purposes for which they were never intended. It is for this reason many have been discredited.

It is important for every individual to be able to understand the workings of their own body and take care of it in the way that benefits that person the most. A good start is by learning to distinguish between sales hype and good sense. Whether the ads are for pharmaceuticals, remedies, supplements to transform the body, or vitamins it is always a good idea to think what the long term effect will be before giving into the latest trends or the next wonder drug just because the person selling it says it is wonderful.

How do you do this? The answer to that question is to think before deciding to try something new, learn how your body truly functions, listen to your own mind and follow intuition and instinct to know what will actually beneficial you. We have learned to do this with used car salesmen—why not where our body is concerned—after all, it is the only model we will ever get.

The first step in sidestepping the sales pitch is to take a moment to recognize the words that should send danger signals. These may include, "all natural is completely safe", "makes you feel young again", "gives you the mental edge you once had", "reverses aging", "you will feel great", etc. The truth is that many supplement products will make you feel younger for a time, but the damage to the overall function of the body will be quicker aging and loss of functions after the glow of newness has warn off. Forcing the body to do age-reversing and cleansing processes against its will is similar to the idea of "succumbing to the dark side" as George Lucas would put it. Many products produce faster and easier results, but they can lead to the shutdown of normal body functions. In fact, many of the "natural" products on the market today have the potential of actually shortening the normal life span.

I began to study homeopathy after my son was given a remedy that allowed him to reverse the effects of autism to become a fully functional, highly intelligent individual. The year was 1982 and I was living in Pakistan. My daughter was able to keep her tonsils in spite of several severe infections and I was able to become truly healthy. It did not matter to me at the time that I had never heard of homeopathy. It did not matter to me that the conventionally trained doctors around me tried to talk me out of using the remedies. I could see the results and I was amazed. I knew instinctively that the promise of no side effects or harm was correct. I knew I could never harm anyone by using these remedies—not my children, not myself and not my clients. That meant a lot to me in the beginning and still does. To affect the health and change problems for anyone without any possibility of harm was the most amazing idea—and I went for it whole heartedly without hesitation.

Over the last twenty three years, I have studied, experimented and continued to apply what I have learned to help many, many people live better lives. If I could not help, at least I have never done any harm. I continue to learn new ways to use this system. One thing I know is that homeopathy contains far more healing potential than I will ever uncover in my lifetime. I truly expect the system for using homeopathy on an energetic level I have developed can continue to uncover ways to heal long after I am gone.

Homeopathy has pervailed over the last 200 years through many trials and changes in attitude, which alone is a testimonial to its efficacy and safety, but the full power of homeopathic healing abilities is yet to be realized.

I have long felt that sitting behind a desk in an office and helping one person at a time as they came through my door was not an efficient method for transforming our current health crisis into healthy living for everyone who will listen. I want you to read what I have learned, whether I ever meet you face to face or not.

Who wants you to be healthy more than you do? The key to your good health lies within your own intuition and good sense. Trust yourself and listen to your heart in order to make the health decisions that will keep you as healthy as you can be.

In the minds of most people in the U.S., homeopathic remedies are grouped in with all other natural supplements such as herbal remedies, flower essences and vitamins. Typically, when I confess to being a homeopathic practitioner, the questions coming fast and furiously are usually questions about herbs. People are stunned when I try to explain that I am not an herbalist. So, what exactly is a homeopathic remedy, you might ask? Indeed, what is a homeopathic remedy? Well, it is not a vitamin, it is not an herb or a magic pill. Yet, homeopathy can do for you what none of these can do. Good health does not come with controlling symptoms, but rather in correcting the underlying problem where the symptoms originate. If you would like to live your life free of problems that lead to pain, depression, compromise in lifestyle, or weight accumulation, read on. Homeopathic remedies are those little bottles or tiny tubes with only sugar pellets inside tucked away behind the counter or in the back of your favorite vitamin or health food store. There is nothing in the bottle except little sugar pills. So, why am I even writing this book? Why are these little tubes and bottles even on the shelf? Because, they really do something to improve the overall health of everyone, in spite of the trashing exposes you've seen on TV or read on the internet lately.

"Thus homeopathy is a perfectly simple system of medicine, remaining always fixed in its principles as in its practice, which, like the doctrine whereon it is based, if rightly apprehended, will be found to be complete (and serviceable)."

Samuel Hahnemann

March 28, 1833

1

A Nutrient Absorption Problem

The human body is made up of billions of tiny biological cells, each alive as a separate entity that eats, metabolizes, excretes, reproduces and dies. Each of these individual cells has requirements of nutrition to keep them healthy and functioning properly. If the inherited code in the cell memory is unable to recognize certain nutrients as good food and something useful, the cell will not take in the food. If a large number of cells in the body fail to recognize a nutrient as necessary, the entire body will feel the stress of deficiency. The fluid between the cells may be awash with these nutrients, but the cells have to take it in and use it on a large scale for the body to be relieved of the stress.

On March 9th 2004, NBC Nightly News® reported America's number one cause of preventable death is obesity and that doctors do not know why Americans are getting fatter and fatter. On Feb. 23, 2004, Time Magazine® published an article "The Silent Killer—Inflammation". The article explains that inflammation is now seen as the cause of stroke and heart disease and that doctors have no clue why chronic inflammation occurs. What is medical research ignoring?

• The Missing Mineral

There is a complex of symptoms that I treat homeopathically more often than any other problem. At least 70% of the people I see in my practice fall into this complex. I believe the reasons are many including immigration of populations from areas where the mineral content in the soil was different than in the U.S. (this is particularly true for the British Isles countries), working under florescent lighting, drinking purified water and the overwhelming use of carbonated drinks in this country. I did not see anywhere near the same number of people with these problems when I practiced in Pakistan. There the population has been homogeneous and indigenous to the area for nearly three thousand years. During the time I lived in Pakistan, there was far less exposure to industry driven environmental issues than we see in the U.S. Soda was a luxury and bottled water was unheard of.

This complex of symptoms is marked by a history of recurring infections, beginning with ear infections in childhood. If it is not ear infections, it is tonsillitis, or bronchitis. Sometimes it is kidney, bladder, upper respiratory, or sinus infections. Whatever the site of infection, it will have been recurring throughout a person's lifetime and chronic inflammation will develop in areas where infection has occurred.

Many people will say "I'm never sick", but closer examination will reveal minor yet definite recurring infections. These may not have been severe enough to put the person in bed, yet the problem may never have been completely relieved or has become chronic. Whatever the infection is, or how severe or minor it may be, there is always a history of infection when this common mineral is missing.

Another problem this person would find is that broken bones and injuries would heal slowly. Maybe this person would be more prone to injury when playing sports than other people, and there would be a tendency for excess scar tissue formation. There has been a report in the news recently that children are suffering broken bones at a rate never seen before. This is one more piece of evidence that this problem with mineral absorption is becoming very widespread.

• Depression

This person will have bouts of depression, perhaps even going back to the teen years. If there is not actual clinical depression, there could be feelings of worthlessness due to low energy levels and feeling as if nothing can ever be accomplished. Perhaps it is a self-esteem problem or a lack of self-confidence. Many times there is seasonal depression. This is the situation where the person gets depressed in the winter when it gets cold and cloudy due to lack of sunlight on the skin and failure to produce or hang on to vitamin D.

I have seen people who were depressed from October when the daylight savings time changes to standard time until March when the time changes back. I may see more people with this condition in Southern California than I would in other parts of the country since so many of the sufferers have moved to Southern California for the sunny climate.

• Sugar Cravings

This person would have a tendency to crave sweets and foods with high sugar content, or stimulants such as coffee, or even diet pills. This is due to the fact that this person's metabolism will be on the lower end of normal and eating sugar gives a temporary lift.

• Poor Muscle Tone

This person will have poor muscle tone. The muscles will be flabby, toneless and exercise will change nothing. Parents and teachers may have verbally abused these people as children for not trying harder, but the person knows attempts to be active yield little or no results.

For this person, activities requiring strength will be completely undoable. As a child and even into adulthood, this person will appear sedentary. Movement is painful, tiresome and worthless. Even the skin will be easily prone to pain--even from minor touch. This could play out in the person avoiding physical contact with other people or not be able to wear tight-fitting clothing.

This person is more likely to be the kind of person who would be easily fatigued when attempting active sports, or be unable to perform certain sports due to poor muscle tone. On the other hand these are the people who can continue low-keyed levels of activity far longer than others since the lack of muscle tone limits the build up of fatigue related chemicals.

• Stomach Acid Imbalance

Other symptoms of this condition could be a life-long problem with improper stomach acidity. This person is prone to heartburn and may develop stomach ulcers or acid reflux disease later in life. Most commonly, the person is always hungry. The high stomach acidity problem creates the situation where food digests faster than a person with a different biochemistry. There is no natural control on eating because the stomach is always empty and burning for more food to calm it down. This is also the person who does not feel satiation when they have had enough to eat and the stomach is full. These people will only stop eating when the belt is tight and the stomach is completely stuffed. There will also be a life-long problem with constipation.

Not all the people I see with this complex of symptoms are terribly overweight, but most are. Some are only slightly overweight and have learned to bypass some of the symptoms enough to control weight to some extent, particularly in the teen years and early twenties. Most, however, will be very overweight or will become more so as they get older.

The weight issue is due to the fact that calcium deficient cells cry out for the nutrient they are not able to get, even where there is over saturation of calories--causing the person to consume beyond need in this vain attempt to be nourished. The blame put forth toward the fast food industry for the fat content of the food being made available to the population of calcium deficient Americans does not address the actual problem. The person suffering from calcium deficiency in the cells of the body has no way to monitor how much they have eaten. The brain never tells them to stop eating because the cells are still trying to get what is missing--and the stomach is always empty and ready for more.

Mostly, people are born with this complex of symptoms. If their parents do not have the same symptoms, a grandparent did. If they did not show the signs of it from childhood, it could have been acquired from accident where many bones were broken--

or from severe head injury. This is because the body's extreme need for calcium to heal head injury or broken bones--or even minor surgery in some cases, puts the rest of the body in calcium deficiency.

The greatest problem facing the American people today is this calcium deficiency. It is the reason adults are fatter than ever. It is the reason kids would rather spend recess eating than playing. It is a condition that is completely undetectable by the technology of medical science. In my opinion, it accounts for a lot of the medical problems we see in today's world that didn't exist forty or fifty years ago—such as high blood pressure, obesity and type 2 diabetes in children. Unusual inflammation in tissues (see Time Magazine, Feb. 23, 2004) and the increase in undetectable heart conditions in adults are also part of this problem. This may be true because the calcium deficiency that our parents displayed slightly is passed on to the next generation of children where it appears in a more severe form. Each generation displaying symptoms of calcium deficiency is more severely affected than the previous generation.

The body can be awash with calcium in the blood stream or in the fluid around tissue due to supplementation, but if the calcium is not passing into the individual cells of the tissues, all the symptoms I describe here will be present. Medical science can only measure the calcium in the blood, not in the tissue. The cells reject the calcium molecule because it is large and looks to be a foreign object to cells where absorption was interrupted due to ongoing stress that has shut down receptor sites, or the deficiency of an accompanying mineral such as iodine.

• Changes

With the use of homeopathically prepared calcium remedies (the Calcarea remedies) all of these symptoms change and the problems disappear.

Calcium is what the body uses to fight infection and kill bacteria through the immune system. Homeopathic Calcarea remedies stop the infections. This includes ear infections in babies and all other recurring infections.

Calcarea remedies stop the heartburn and stomach symptoms by stabilizing calcium in the digestive tract and balancing the level of acidity.

Calcarea remedies have an impact on the metabolism. I have seen children who couldn't do anything but watch TV everyday after school get up and go out to play almost immediately after beginning a regime of homeopathic Calcarea remedies. A child without calcium absorption problems won't stay inside or remain inactive. In addition to becoming more physically active, these children begin to be more interested in school and show a rise in self-confidence. Older clients report the same increase in interest in their job or school activity, a desire for increased physical activity and the disappearance of depression or the need to be in the sun all year around.

With calcium absorption, muscle tone improves. Incorrect calcium absorption causes nerve endings to fire off incorrectly creating a lack of muscle tone--including the muscle structure of blood vessels. Lack of calcium causes an integrity problem in the circulatory systems of the body.

The use of homeopathically prepared calcium helps the calcium molecule begin to fill into the cells of muscle tissue. Muscles begin to develop tone and blood vessels improve integrity. This process can take a bit of time. When it happened to me, I felt a ring of tone begin at the base of my legs and move up through the muscles as if the ring were being pulled upward. My muscles became firm, but it took about a year. Many people report a loss of inches during this process without a loss of weight. This is because the muscles and bones are gaining weight in density that is being converted from fat. One becomes slim, but it is not apparent on the scales.

By balancing calcium, injuries do not occur easily--and if they do, they heal quickly. It becomes more comfortable for the individual to move around and exercise, and exercise is more effective in producing weight loss and muscle tone. People who are athletic and have always had good muscle tone would never have experienced any of the symptoms of this complex.

A homeopathic regime of Calcarea and other calcium absorption remedies will change all of the symptoms, but the situation does not change permanently without dietary supplementation of elemental calcium---nor does calcium absorb correctly without the use of the homeopathic forms. This is true because the homeopathic diluted form of calcium teaches the cells of the tissues to absorb the calcium molecule, which the cell perceived as too large and too foreign after absorption was interrupted at some time in the past. The cells learn to absorb and the symptoms go away. However, these symptoms do not continue to stay away unless actual material doses of calcium are provided.

If a person with this complex takes calcium as a material mineral dietary supplement, none of the symptoms would go away because the tissues would still not be absorbing calcium. Homeopathic calcium remedies teach the cells to absorb, but do not provide calcium for them to absorb. Only a combination of the homeopathic form in conjunction with the dietary material supplement will work.

• Change Takes Time

Remember, we are talking of permanent changes in body type and function. This is a change that takes time and patience. If you want the changes, you must realize it takes a few remedies and a certain amount of time. Many changes will be apparent immediately, but this does not mean one stops taking the remedy. The full extent of the changes will not be apparent right away, but how long changes will continue depends on the situation of each individual. The good news is that regardless of diet, lifestyle and environmental factors changes and good health do occur.

• Calcarea is Latin for Calcium

All homeopathic remedies are written in Latin to distinguish them from pharmaceuticals and herbs. The Calcarea remedies are derived from calcium and converted to energy by dilution and succession. The Calcarea remedies describe all the symptoms of the lack of calcium problem and, therefore, relieve all of those problems. The complete list of Calcarea related symptoms can be found in the <u>Handbook of Homeopathic Materia Medica with Repertory</u> by William Boericke.

• In the News

Early in 2004, a story hit the news concerning new research that had identified a link between the extensive use of antibiotics and the occurrence of breast cancer. Suddenly, everyone who had used antibiotics was afraid they had done something to compromise their health.

Upon hearing this news, my first thought was that although scientists had identified a link, the blame placed on antibiotics as a cause of breast cancer was a misinterpretation of the data. It is much more reasonable to suspect that the overall health pattern of the individual that creates the need for the antibiotics is also the factor that leaves the person prone to develop cancer because of a poor immune system. In other words, people who are calcium deficient have more recurring infections, more need for antibiotics and an immune system that probably has trouble holding back the uncontrolled growth of cancerous cells.

I saw an article in the "San Bernardino Sun Newspaper" in the March 6th 2004 edition. In this article, two leading medical groups are said to be recommending that doctors stop treating childhood ear infections with antibiotic, as the article put it, "leaving parents with whimpering, infected toddlers and no alternative." Although the article did not say why these medical groups are recommending this approach, it seems obvious the fears concerning the over-use of antibiotics must be a factor.

Recurring ear infections in children is one of the common symptoms of calcium absorption problems. I have seen this problem cleared up many, many times, maybe hundreds of time by the use of homeopathic Calcarea remedies in conjunction with small amounts of supplemented calcium. If the child is very young, there is no need for calcium supplementation. The homeopathic remedy Calc. Phos. 6X can clear this problem of recurring ear infections without any help from a supplement or additional remedy.

I once asked my mother what the world had been like before the days of antibiotics. "Didn't a lot of people die of infections?" I asked.

"It wasn't that bad," she answered. "People didn't seem to get infections in those days like they do now."

Many experts have blamed the use of the antibiotics for developing a need and dependence on the drug. I disagree. The way I see it, antibiotics were developed just at the time the problem of calcium deficiency began to be a problem--just as the baby boomer generation was being born. This generation was born just after the stress of the greatest war ever, to parents who were children of immigrants from places in the world where the soils and food supply was rich in iodine from sea water infusion or kelp fertilization causing an iodine deficiency, thyroid hormonal slow down and, therefore, calcium absorption interruption that is intensifying from one generation to the next. In my opinion, this is the reason why Americans are the fattest nation on earth and the largest consumers of antibiotics. The fact that most people are totally clueless to the dynamics of this problem is leading to a health crisis never before seen in history.

2

The Cinderella Factor

The story of the little cinder girl rising above adverse conditions and her dreary life to marry the handsome prince is a story that has captured our imagination for centuries. I alone can remember at least ten different movie and television productions of this timeless story.

Why does it have such an appeal to us? Why do we continue to enjoy a good Cinderella story?

I once had an argument with a college professor during a time I was taking classes for teacher credentialing. She had built a career and a lifestyle on the idea that Cinderella represented a young girl who had been raised from her dreary background not by her own ambitions or integrity, but only by marriage to the prince. In her opinion, it was marriage to the prince that created and defined the role of Cinderella. Oddly, I don't remember any of the stories continuing on to reveal Cinderella's role as a princess.

I suggested she look again. The story of Cinderella appeals to us because it represents a young girl who was able to raise herself above her petty, working class, corrupt, downtrodden surroundings and background to achieve the highest position possible in the land. She did this remarkable thing by her own integrity, kindness, intelligence and belief in herself. The prince fell in love with her because she possessed all of the qualities he admired, not because his attention created her abilities. The message here is that Cinderella represents someone who can achieve greatness no matter where she has come from. That is an inspiration to all of us.

So, you may ask, why am I telling this story in a book about homeopathic remedies? For this simple reason—no matter where our parents or ancestors immigrated from--no matter our physical or cultural heritage--no matter how hurt we feel by our present status or our physical condition, homeopathy is our fairy godmother. We can rise above our past to achieve the most optimum level possible in physical and mental function.

Homeopathy is not super nutrition. It will not make you superman. It will help you achieve all that is possible for you. The Cinderella effect of homeopathy means that it is possible to rise above your insecure, petty, manipulative, controlling relatives—who only do these things out of fear and their own insecurities—to become whatever you wish to become. Cinderella's step mother and sisters only suppressed her and treated her badly out of fear of her special-ness and natural abilities.

It is possible to rise above fear, shame, anger and the hold the past has on us to a position where our special-ness can shine through. Never doubt that you are Cinderella underneath the cinders.

• Self-esteem

Problems with a person's feelings of worth are not always problems stemming from environment. Many times problems with self-esteem stem from calcium deficiency problems as we talked about in the last chapter. If a person's basic organism is deficient in the basic minerals necessary for proper function, it is natural for the entire organism to react in ways that would prevent the person from putting themselves into positions of vulnerability. In our society, this unwillingness to go ahead with the next step, or move forward, or begin a new project appears as a problem with a person's feeling of worth. In reality, it is a problem with basic brain chemistry which renders a person in need of alternate routes to achieve everyday goals.

One example of the manifestation of a brain chemistry problem that translates into what appears as a social problem can be associated with the adolescent girl who stops being a good student at the age of 12 or 13 and begins to be interested in boys. I have heard this problem described many times by parents and teachers. I have known teachers who knew female students in the fifth grade and described these girls as brilliant, straight A students and very good at math who became sixth grade students that displayed none of these qualities.

What took place between the fifth and sixth grades to change these good students into girls who begin to take on friendships with boy? Many educators have often expressed a belief that it is a socialization problem at the time students are going through puberty and beginning to notice the opposite sex. But is it really? Do girls suddenly want to appear dumb in order to attract the attention of boys as many teachers believe? In fact, what actually does occur is the onset of the menstrual cycle. In many girls, particularly girls with the disposition to be calcium deficient, the onset of the monthly menstrual cycle means that iron is lost through blood loss each month. It should not be this way, but very commonly is. As girls lose iron, the brain loses iron as a chemical necessary to do math and other calculating skills. Boys mature more slowly and over a longer period of time. Boys never develop an iron losing cycle and never lose an ability to do math if they had the ability in the earlier grades. The female desire to hang around boys may be an attempt to pick up a skill that has been lost that remains intact in the opposite sex. Using homeopathic prepared Ferrum remedies in high potencies for mental development is a way to bring math ability back to girls who display a problem after puberty. (more on this later)

Self-esteem problems may also appear as shyness. A person who is calcium and copper deficient has a very difficult time judging how they relate to other people. Just as the character of Phoebe on the television show "Friends" does not know how bad she is at singing and playing the guitar, many people do not know if people like them, if what they say is appropriate, or even if people are laughing at them or not. In this stage of uncertainty, it is much easier to avoid social situations than to try and understand how one actually relates to the world. Calcium and copper in homeopathic forms can clear these problems, allowing the person to be all that they can be and achieve all that is possible for them to achieve.

• Excess Weight

Many of you know what someone means when they say, "I just can't lose weight no matter how much I starve myself and exercise."

Many of you know what it's like to gain weight and be fat on a diet that keeps other people at a normal weight.

Many of you know the mental anguish of constantly having to think about control.

Many of you know what exercising and seeing no results feels like.

Many of you know what it feels like to not be believed and have people say, "but you must be doing something to make yourself fat, flabby, and unattractive."

Many of you know that dieting only brings on more weight.

No one wants to be a hundred pounds overweight. When slim, firm bodied people work out, they get results. Slim people don't think about food and control, it just happens--and it has always been that way. When people who are prone to weight gain lose weight, it is a matter of intense control and is always temporary. If slim people gain a few pounds, a good work out and a few days of dieting put things right again. It is not lifestyle that makes the difference, no matter what the experts say.

I believe people when they say they really don't eat much and are still fat. I know how it feels to have people believe you are a closet binger.

I believe people who say they just can't lose weight.

I believe because I've been one of them all of my life.

I was put on diets by doctors from as early an age as I can remember. I had a metabolism test when I was in the second grade. I was put on diet supplements and powdered meals in grammar school. There were more metabolism tests, thyroid hormones and amphetamines in high school. This was during the amphetamine culture of the 1960's and the drug was prescribed by a doctor who thought he was doing the right thing. I felt a rush for a few days, lost my appetite for about a week, but didn't lose any weight. We now know stimulants and anything that works like an amphetamine does not work for long and weight comes right back. By the time I was eighteen, I had tried it all and I was fatter than ever.

While I was attending college, I fell into a life style where I didn't eat for several days at a time. Often I would eat only 2 or 3 meals a week. I was walking constantly across a very large campus, and still, after an entire year of living this way, I had only managed to lose 20 pounds. For a person without a weight problem, anorexia could have been suspect. Yet, I was still thirty pounds overweight. I was still flabby. My muscles were soft and toneless. My husband commented on this shortly after we were married.

When my children were born, I experienced several bouts of recurring infections ranging from breast infections (mastitis) to kidney infections and several root canal treatments due to dental infections. It seemed I was always on antibiotics.

As my children grew, they were not overweight, since they were their father's children, but they did suffer from infections. It was in a desperate attempt to solve the infections that I was first introduced to homeopathic remedies.

Homeopathy was remarkable for stopping the infections and transforming our lives and I was fascinated by it from the moment I first discovered it.

From the beginning, I had one goal in mind above all others. From my study, practice and experimentation with homeopathy, I had to find a solution to the weight problem. There were some remedies mentioned in the literature and I tried them all, but nothing held for me. There had to be other factors. I was always convinced that someday I would find an answer in homeopathy. The answer is the absorption of calcium and the balancing of insulin in the cells of the body. Only homeopathy can make this change. After all of these years, I have finally found the key and the answer to this problem that plagues more Americans than the citizens of any other nation on the planet.

• Supplements are Not All Wonderful

For a period of about five years, I worked at a homeopathic pharmacy in West Hollywood as a homeopathic consultant. During this time, I became familiar with a lot of over-the-counter products and supplements. One thing I came to know is that not all dietary supplements are actually good for the body—mainly because people take more than the body can handle. This is also true of herbs. In general, if an herb had never been used as a food or used on a continuous basis in the indigenous culture where it originated, it is very likely to cause side effects if it is overused. Herbs are chemical based medicines. Natural and legal does not mean harmless. Mu Huang, or Ephedra, is not only dangerous for its heart stimulating effect, but weight that is lost with it will always come back. It is now controlled by law. The effect of any stimulant, even ginseng, on the body is exactly the same as that of amphetamines. I have seen it over and over. When people lose weight with a stimulant, the weight comes right back.

- ## Failed Diet Products

In recent years, many diet-aid products have hit the dietary supplement industry. These products would come into the pharmacy with lots of hype and fan fare. People would rush in to buy them and the store would run out. In the next round the ordering department would order larger quantities and there they would sit. The people who bought the first round never returned to buy more.

Just as with amphetamines, the use of a metabolism stimulant will appear to work in the beginning and some weight will be lost. However, the weight will always come back. This is because the use of a stimulant has the effect of disconnecting the physical body from the mental realms. When this happens, the person loses a feeling for what they have eaten and begins to eat more than they would have before this experience. Also, stimulants shut down receptor sites where nutrients are taken into individual cells, causing cells to metabolize less nutrients and the body to store more of what is eaten as fat. This happens with any stimulant product.

- ## Too Many Minerals

In recent years, several magazine articles have been published that suggest the common mineral calcium can be an aid to weight loss--particularly for women. Many doctors have suggested their patients take supplements of calcium for general health and to stop the onset of osteoporosis. I have known for some time that many people who have taken high doses of calcium for a while can suffer from a new problem caused by accumulation of calcium in the inter-cellular fluids because the body is often unable to throw off the excess, causing bone spurs and fibroid tumors. The homeopathic form of calcium, Calcarea, will make sure cells absorb calcium correctly, eliminating the excess where it should not be and encouraging receptor sites on cells to absorb more calcium--which improves metabolism, muscle tone and satiation response.

Many people who have had stomach surgery to reduce the appetite will eventually begin to gain the weight back. This is sometimes due to the fact that internal cellular mineral absorption problems have not changed and the body still demands the nutrient it cannot absorb, therefore, the appetite remains high as lifestyle increases the stomach capacity. Since muscle tone and appetite have not changed, the results changed by surgery will only be temporary.

The proper absorption of calcium is very helpful in reducing and stabilizing weight for most people who have the symptoms talked about in Chapter 1. However, there is another situation which is far more difficult to handle. This situation is now called Metabolic disorder, Syndrome X, or insulin resistance disorder and is usually seen in people over forty years of age, who may or may not have a history of diabetes in their family, but carry their weight in the upper part of the body, particularly in the abdomen. If you fall into this category and find weight very difficult or impossible to lose, it is because your body has created this problem in response to your use of stimulants to lose weight in the past, or because you have suffered through an ongoing emotional stress situation that created the same effect-- permanent weight gain.

What follows in this book is the complete story of homeopathy, its history and the true nature of how it works. You will read about calcium and how homeopathy can solve many problems that we as human beings are prone to and need to address--including weight problems and insulin resistance.

3

Homeopathy in the U.S.

A question frequently asked by people when first presented with the idea of using homeopathic remedies as a form of medical treatment or for the correction of chronic problems is, "If it is so good, how come I'd never heard of it before now?"

For those with a slight understanding of the history of medicine in the United States, the question often arises, "If homeopathy works and is so valuable, what factors allowed it to disappear so completely from the U.S. in the 1920's?" Both of these questions are valid and it is only by a careful study of the history and politics of that time that one is able to determine how and why the homeopathic field was lost from the American consciousness.

• During the Civil War

The demise of homeopathy in American has its roots in the Civil War. The Civil War affected Americans in many ways not limited to the battlefield casualties. Large groups of men were gathered together for the first time in U.S. history and mass epidemics of diseases such as measles, chickenpox and other "childhood" ailments swept through the ranks and the country side. Prior to this time, the isolating effects of the agricultural community limited these outbreaks to the cities where strict quarantine laws controlled their spread.

These events, ironically, actually began the growth of the homeopathic industry because homeopathy offered some relief of the symptoms of these diseases in this pre-antibiotic era. Unfortunately, battlefield casualties did not respond to homeopathic treatment and it was the actual war that fostered the growth of allopathic medical specialties such as surgery, pharmaceuticals for pain control and surgical anesthesia.

• Homeopathy and Allopathy Together

The division between these two branches of medicine, Homeopathy and Allopathy (conventional medicine), continued, but each had a profound respect for the other. It was common for a physician to be trained both in the homeopathic and allopathic fields. It was not unusual for physicians to freely consult with any practitioner in an attempt to find any possible way to help their patients.

In general, practitioners and the public as a whole did not believe there to be any superiority which would rank one system above the other. Each system had its individual supporters who insisted theirs was the only system that should be used. However, the rivalry was more on a "sports match" basis where people preferred their particular division of medicine the same way people now prefer the Cubs or the Yankees, always insisting that for this particular disease theirs was the best and would "win".

• The First World War Brought Changes

It was the advent of the First World War that proved to be the decisive factor in the United States. During World War I, the massive movement of people and soldiers back and forth to other countries resulted in pandemics of Influenza and other diseases. The battlefield injuries along with these new diseases created conditions and illnesses that the slower effects of homeopathic remedies could not handle. As it became apparent at that time, allopathic techniques were better equipped to handle acute care of highly infectious diseases and life-threatening injuries, such as those caused by war. The demise of homeopathy in America began as fear of future wars drove the government to back a system that could keep soldiers on the field and support laborers in the work force. The American Medical Association was formed and the homeopathic schools were shut down or converted to allopathic institutions.

It should be noted that other countries more directly affected by the war did not drop homeopathy from their medical systems. There are several reasons why homeopathy remained a viable and respected form of medicine in these other countries. For the most part, other countries had never created a complete division between the two modalities as had occurred in the U.S. during the Civil War. After World War I, America entered a period of isolationism and believed that by limiting access to its shores, it could prevent the massive epidemics which continued to sweep through other less isolated countries.

From an economic stand point, America had prospered during the war, where other countries, in which the battles were actually fought, suffered massive devastation and could not afford the high cost associated with pure allopathic treatment. In these countries, homeopathy was valued for its safety, efficacy and low cost. Even after these war-ravaged economies began to recover from the devastation caused by the war, homeopathy was valued as a low cost, highly effective form of preventive medicine and obtained a degree of respect and acceptance in the allopathic communities.

Politically, Americans began to look to their government for means by which "big industry" could be kept honest. Divisions in the government, such as the Department of Agriculture, created to oversee the purity of the food producing industries, and the Food and Drug Administration, created to oversee the purity of processed foods, the cleanliness of restaurants and eating establishments, along with the efficacy and purity of the pharmaceutical industries, were among some of the many agencies created to assure the safety of the consumer. Because homeopathic medicines cannot be chemically analyzed, there was no way the FDA could determine their purity. From a chemical standpoint, all homeopathic medicines are identical and equivalent to common table sugar.

• Resurgence of Interest

All of these and other factors resulted in the state of medical technologies as it exists today. But it is the dissatisfaction of the consumer that has led to the world-wide search for other healing modalities. In America today, there is a resurgence of the previously shunned art of homeopathy along with the emergence of Traditional Chinese Medicine and the healing arts normally associated with Eastern Cultures. This increasingly wider range of modalities has allowed the consumer a wide variety of options by which personal control over their bodies and their personal health and well being can be exercised.

4

Where Homeopathy Began

Samuel Hahnemann was born on April 10th, 1755 at Meissen, in Saxony, Germany. He was the son of an Artisan, a porcelain painter. His childhood was humble, and he attended Meissen High School by becoming a servant in the house of one of the masters. Hahnemann received a classical education, and was a top student in the languages of Greek and Latin.

In 1775, at the age of twenty, Hahnemann started his studies of medicine in Leipsic. He made his living by giving instruction in German and French and by translating English books into German. In 1779, he received a degree as an M.D.

In 1782, Hahnemann took the post of parish doctor in Dessau, met Johanna Kuchler and married. On beginning to practice his profession, Hahnemann wrote that there had previously been no physician at this place, and that the inhabitants had no desire for any such person. He remained there two and half years and commented that the people probably would have done quite well without him.

• Hahnemann Quits Medicine

In 1784, Hahnemann gave up the practice of medicine entirely, explaining that the rude and barbarous medical methods of the day disturbed his logical and educated mind, which was trained to expect definite results. He disliked giving compounds, the effects of which were unknown. He explained that he could not accept the loose ways and methods of the existing medical schools, hampered by dogmas of doubt and uncertainty. He could no longer accept the risk of doing injury and turned to chemistry and translation as a means of livelihood.

The family moved to Dresden, where Hahnemann translated and studied chemistry and medical jurisprudence. He was accepted among the scholars of the city and became known as a scholarly man among them.

In September, 1789, the family moved to Leipzig where Hahnemann continued his literary work.

Because of his literary work and translation of medical text, Hahnemann would most certainly have been familiar with Stahl's doctrine of the "vital force" popular in France at the time.

However, it was while translating from English the materia medica of the Scottish physician, William Cullen, that Hahnemann discovered statements which spoke about a 'nervous energy' as the determinant of the normal state of the body. It is likely that the synthesis of these two ideas led to the beginning of homeopathic theory. Hahnemann began his exploration of this new concept by conducting the original experiments on himself. He wrote:

> I took by way of experiment, twice a day four drachmas, of good China (Peruvian Bark). My feet and finger tips at first became cold; I grew languid and drowsy; then my pulse grew hard and small; intolerable anxiety, trembling and prostration throughout all my limbs; then pulsation in my head, redness of my cheeks, thirst and --in short- -all these symptoms which are ordinarily characteristic of Intermittent Fever (Malaria) made their appearance, one after another, yet without the peculiar chilly rigor. This paroxysm lasted two or three hours each time, and recurred if I repeated the dose, not otherwise. I discontinued it and was in good health.

During Hahnemann's time, China (Peruvian Bark) was a common treatment for the disease of Malaria. By taking the cure for a disease not present in the body, Hahnemann was able to observe that the cure would create in a healthy body the same symptoms it would cure in a diseased body. From this breakthrough, Hahnemann developed the concept of "like cures like" and the equally important concept of "proving". That is, administering a substance to a healthy individual in order to "prove" which symptoms it would create, and therefore, would cure.

Hahnemann passed the next six years in experimenting with himself and his family, proving the effects of remedies and recording what he found, eventually using his findings on sick people.

In 1796, in <u>The Journal for Practicing Physicians</u>, the most important medical journal of that time, he published his essay, "A New Principle for Ascertaining the Curative Powers of Drugs". In this article, he first explained the principle of "Like cures Like", declaring that whatever a drug would cause, it would cure.

Between 1799 and 1811, Hahnemann and his family were impoverished, persecuted, and driven from town to town by physicians and apothecaries who accused him of using unfair practices, secret remedies, and quackery.

Hahnemann's first collection of provings was published in Latin in 1805. Five years later the first edition of <u>Organon of the Medical Arts</u> appeared. In this he carefully explained his new medical discoveries and beliefs, mentioning the word Homeopathy for the first time. In the introduction, Hahnemann writes a scathing review of the medical practices of his day by stating that:

--since a time soon after Hippocrates, men have occupied themselves with the treatment of disease while being led astray by their vanity, and by guess work, to devise innumerable and dissimilar ideas about how to treat disease. The systems and structures having risen from so many dissimilar brains and theoretical views, that each is in variance with the rest and self-contradictory. Each of these subtle expositions at first threw the readers into stupefied amazement at the incomprehensible wisdom contained in it, and attracted to the system monger a number of followers, who re-echoes his unnatural sophistry, to none of whom, however, was it of the slightest use in enabling them to cure better, until a new system, often diametrically opposed to the first thrust that aside. None of them was in agreement with nature and experience. They were mere theoretical webs constructed by cunning intellects out of pretended consequences which could not be made use of in practice, in the treatment at the sick-bed, on account of their excessive subtlety and repugnance to nature and only served for empty disputations. Simultaneously, but quite independent of all these theories, there sprang up a mode of treatment with mixtures of unknown medicinal substances, against forms of disease arbitrarily set up, and directed towards some material object completely at variance with nature and experience, hence, as may be supposed, with a bad result--such is old medicine, Allopathy as it is termed.

Hahnemann's new philosophy was a return to the teaching of Hippocrates which emphasized the need to observe the condition of the patient and make inquiries into all aspects of the illness. Due to the concept of "like cures like", it was extremely important to gather all symptoms present in a condition in order that the proper remedy could be determined.

• Vital Force

In his book, <u>Organon of Medicine</u>, Hahnemann explained that there is a vital force, a non-material entity that governs the material body. According to his concepts, it is not the body that is ill, but rather the vital force that has been disrupted and thrown out of balance. Disease is not what makes a person sick, it is a breakdown in the body's energy or vital force that allows disease causing entities to enter the energy bodies of the individual and create the symptoms that are observed. One cannot bring about a cure by treating the body on only the chemical level, but rather by using a substance, potentized to an energy level (Chapters 6 & 7). It is the administration of this energy to the sick individual --thereby treating the energy body (or vital force) in a non-invasive, non-harmful manner which allows the health to be restored.

• Do No Harm

Hahnemann followed Hippocrates' dictum, "above all else, the physician should do no harm". Hahnemann noted that diluted and potentized substances lacked the ability to do harm to the physical body and were a safe alternative to the healing practices of the day. As he further diluted and succussed his remedies, Hahnemann discovered that not only did the remedy become safer on a physical level, but also became stronger on a curative level. It was by successive dilutions, potentizing and experimentation that Hahnemann created the range of curative potencies so familiar with today's practitioners. Adherence to these concepts and practices are the foundations that make homeopathy an accepted alternative (natural) healing system wherever and however it is practiced in the world today. It is a fact that in today's world, homeopathy is practiced in a variety of ways, using many varied levels of potency.

Hahnemann's philosophy was in great contrast to the allopathic medical practices of his day where drastic, painful and harmful physical procedures were common. This difference alone could have accounted for the great success Hahnemann found in his later years as a famous and much sought after healer entrenched in upper class Parisian society of the mid-nineteenth century. Yet, in addition to the use of painless methods, he was able to make some amazing cures, using remedies he made himself, and experimenting with different ways of using potencies.

Hahnemann had many students who learned his philosophy and methods and later went out into the world to practice and acquire students of their own. Some made adjustments to the original methods to fit the situations they found themselves facing. Some seemed to cling tenaciously to Hahnemann's early methods even as the master himself was changing. Some learned Hahnemann's newer methods and ignored earlier teachings, creating additional schools of thought. Throughout the two centuries that have elapsed, the word homeopathy has become host to many practices that have developed into different schools claiming allegiance to some original Hahnemannian method or to various historic figures who interpreted the writings of the founder. It is an amazing feature of the system that even used in a variety of methods homeopathy can help bring the human body to balance and health.

• The True Nature of Energy

The school that comes closest to the true nature of "classical" homeopathy is the American school as it existed in the 1920's, sometimes called the Kentian school, after James T. Kent, one of homeopathy's greatest teachers. The practice of classical homeopathy is more than an adherence to the methods of a particular school; it is adherence to the true nature of energy and the laws that govern energy's effect on the non-material parts of the human being.

Medical science has, as yet, been unable to prove the existence of all the energy levels that will be discussed in this book. Although studies such as Kirlian photography and electro acupuncture have proven the existence of previously unknown aspects of the body's energy fields, medical science today still struggles with these concepts.

Homeopathy in the Twentieth Century

In the late Nineteenth and early Twentieth Century, there were over 20 medical schools in America dedicated to the teaching of homeopathy. These supplied the homeopathic practitioners for more than 100 homeopathic hospitals and utilized the services of more than 1,000 homeopathic pharmacies. In 1900, the U.S. was considered the world leader in homeopathy. The best homeopathic doctors in the world either taught or were trained in the United States. These included William Boericke who taught and lectured at the University of California, and James T. Kent who taught at the Hahnemann College in Philadelphia. Homeopathy was more popular in the U.S. than anywhere else in the world.

In the 1920's, the competition between the two

branches of medicine, homeopathy and allopathy, came to a climactic state. For a brief time, it was unclear whether both schools could continue to exist as equals. The American Medical Association (AMA) was a newly formed body and gained some very powerful and wealthy converts. The AMA increased its influence rapidly. Although originally accepting the homeopathic doctors as members, the AMA later forced them to give up their homeopathic licensing and convert to allopathy or cease practicing medicine all together. This set the stage for what many have called the dark ages of homeopathy in the United States. During this time, the homeopathic medical schools were closed and the teaching of homeopathy all but abandoned. Although the pharmacies and book publishers remained in business for a time, most selling their products to foreign countries, many did not survive this period.

The 1970's and 80's brought back a resurgence of interest in the healing powers of homeopathy. In 1989 homeopathic remedies were removed from the list of "by prescription only" drugs and made available "over the counter" for the first time. Unfortunately, largely due to the lack of proper training institutions, homeopathy in America is often a self-taught best-guess system. Although there has recently been a resurgence of classically trained homeopathic practitioner, there remains a segment of the homeopathic community whose adherence to limited interpretations of homeopathic theories become the foundation for the variety of schools we see in the U.S. today.

• Synopsis of Systems

One system teaches its practitioners to use only low potencies, 6's and 9's, given regularly over long periods of time, rarely venturing into the 30's, and calculating exactly how much of the original substance remains, as if its curing power were in the chemical substance and not in the potentized form.

Another system advocates using only a single 200th potency dose and waiting months to see the eventual outcome before suggesting a second potency.

Still another employs doses of very high potencies of 10,000 or more, even repeated frequently over a long period of time.

All of these systems have experienced a degree of success at certain times, or they would not have prevailed, but none can be considered correct for all patients at all times. Although homeopathy cannot physically harm anyone by the use of an inappropriate potency, it can fail to work, thereby, leading the person to believe that homeopathy is ineffective. The wrong potency will result in the remedy not working as desired or producing effects that may not last. It is impossible to get a permanent amelioration of symptoms with a potency that does not reach to the right level.

The best approach is to have the skill and knowledge to use high, medium and low potencies when appropriate according to the signs and needs of the individual. Adherence to the energy body model and the correct use of potency according to the model is the approach that provides the most predictable and consistent results.

In the present climate of growing mistrust and dwindling services, many people now desire to know more about preventive health methods and simple ways to stay healthy. It is possible for the individual to understand the true nature of the body and the energy that controls the physical body in order to use homeopathy effectively for ones own health and well being. Repair of damage, reversal of life-threatening illness and the need for symptom controlling drugs will always remain the work of the conventional medical systems, but preventive maintenance and simple reversal of mineral absorption problems to restore good health can certainly be handled by the individual for themselves and their families. Read on to discover how.

5

The Nature of Energy

The idea that the life force of a person consists mainly of energy is not a new one. The belief that this life force controls the body and can continue outside the material body is a concept found in all cultures from ancient times to the present. At different times and in different cultures, this energy has been called by a variety of names, but the basic concept that an energy force surrounds, penetrates, animates and controls the material body remains consistent. It is only the question of how this force maintains good health and the best methods for correcting disturbances in this vital force that remains in dispute.

• What is Qi?

In Chinese thought from ancient times to the present,

Qi (chi) is the name given to the energy force which penetrates all matter and all living things. Qi is the only substance that possesses force or energy in the universe. At the very birth of the universe there was only Qi. Because of the function and movement of Qi, nature developed in the universe—as did the earth, man and everything else. All are interrelated, interacted, interchanged and interdependent.

The universal energy, Qi, is everything. As the result of Qi, man is a microcosm of the universe. In man all aspects of the universe are reflected and displayed. The vital force of the universe is Qi—the vital force of man is Qi. The universe has spirit, so does man. The earth consists mostly of water, so does man. The universe has the sun, the moon, rain and thunder while man has eyes, tears and voice. The earth can be polluted and sick, so can man. The universe needs the balance and harmony of Qi to function. Both the universe and man obey the same laws.

In Traditional Chinese medicine, it is believed that life is the result of Qi. Without Qi there is no life. The original Qi is given to the body at the point of conception. This original Qi, or vital force, allows the body of the fetus to develop. After birth, the body continues to accumulate Qi by carrying on normal life functions. Qi is brought into the body by breathing air, eating food, absorbing light and moving through the environment.

Qi travels in special channels known as meridians throughout the body. It is stored in the Qi-cavities, but this fact is not noted by conventional medicine. Every illness can be attributed to the improper function or distribution of the various types of Qi. It is the proper balance, distribution and use of this Qi, or vital force, that enables the machinery of the mind-body to function.

In the course of a lifetime, one's mind-body is constantly influenced by every aspect of changing nature, such as weather, geographic location, the seasons, temperature, color, food and emotion. The circulation of Qi can also be influenced by these same phenomena. As a result, this vital force may periodically need "tuning up". Without proper maintenance, the Qi can become stagnant, deficient, excessive, or improperly balanced— all of which allow disease to occur.

Traditional Chinese medicine employs several techniques to correct problems in the Qi. Acupuncture and Qi Gong function as the two main tools for "tuning up" the Qi.

Qi Gong is the ancient Chinese art of creating, manipulating and maintaining the Qi by use of specific exercises that coordinate and develop the mind, breath and body. The goal of Qi Gong is to create smooth functioning of the organism and a state of dynamic equilibrium within the body. This state of equilibrium, or balance, will create well-being in mind and body, prevent disease, relieve sickness, and prolong life.

In Traditional Chinese medicine, acupuncture is the most common method by which Qi is corrected after disharmony or disease has occurred. Acupuncture uses very fine needles which are inserted into specific points along the meridians to reestablish and balance the flow of Qi. When the Qi has returned to its balanced state of equilibrium, the diseases which occurred as a result of the disharmony are reversed. Qi Gong maintains the function of Qi. Acupuncture corrects disharmonies within the Qi.

• The Aura

Today, the science of metaphysics refers to the energy that animates the material body simply as the Aura. Evidence of the Aura has been photographed using special techniques which result in the light-filled energy force being made visible on a photographic print. These photographs depict the variously colored field which surrounds each living being and have been used by certain branches of alternative healing as a diagnostic tool where the color and shape of the Aura are reported to have special meaning. However, one should be aware that while the photograph may show the Aura, the interpretations implied are those of the practitioner and may not be reflected in other branches of alternative healing. The Aura of each individual is unique in frequency and no two people are entirely alike. The Auric fields of one individual interact with those of other people.

Every time a person comes in contact with another person or other living being, an interaction can occur. This interaction can also occur between elements of nature, animals, plants or minerals. The changes in the Aura reflect the physical, emotional, mental and spiritual aspects of the individual. It is the Auric reaction to disease and trauma that is important in the use of homeopathic remedies.

• Energy Bodies

There is general agreement in the alternative medicine world that there are energy bodies which surround each and every living being. The Aura is actually comprised of bands of energy that form distinct bodies. These are bands of energy of varying intensity that surround and interpenetrate the physical body. Their predominant function is to help coordinate and regulate the spirit's activities in physical life. Some of these energy fields (energy bodies) reside within the physical body while others reside and surround the person external to the physical body. It is those outside the physical body that are perceived in the photographs of the Aura.

• The Spirit and Energy Bodies

A distinction has to be made between the soul or spirit of the person and the energy bodies seen in the Aura. The energy bodies are present only in physical life. Their function is to regulate development and allow the individual soul to interact with the body. This is accomplished by bridging the realms between energy and matter. The energy bodies are present from conception, but vanish after death. They do not exist separate from the physical body as the spirit may.

• How Energy Bodies Function

There can be as many as 12 distinguishable energy bodies. They are actually separate layers of energy and have separate functions. The first four develop between conception and birth, and must be present for a living child to be born. Any living being has the first four energy bodies. Their function is in the realm of the development of the physical body, and their presence allows the individual to develop control over the physical body. Disharmonies and disruptions in these first four energy fields will result in various types of birth defects and developmental abnormalities

• Through Age

At different stages and ages through a person's development, other energy bodies develop for different needs. The fifth, the first that is located outside the physical body, has to do with needs and the ability to acquire the means to fulfill the needs by the individual. The sixth is associated with social development, the seventh with knowledge, the eighth with perceptual comprehension, the ninth with the ability to develop awareness of the feelings of others and the tenth with extra-sensory-perception. Individuals differ in the degree to which each of these energy bodies develop, and accordingly, function differently in the associated areas which that body controls. The final two are the last to form and actually function to help the individual prepare to die and make the transition to the next world.

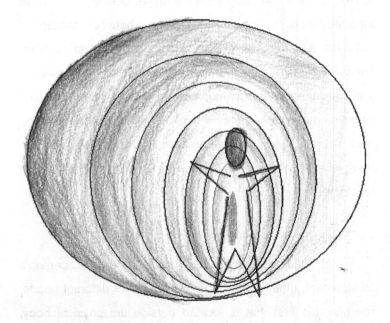

Figure 5:1 A human being is more energy than material substance. The Aura consists of bands of energy bodies.

• Energy Levels

A second very important concept that must be understood when talking about energetic systems is the concept of levels. There are six main levels which, in order, are: 1) physical, 2) mental, 3) emotional, 4) psychological, 5) psychic, 6) spiritual.

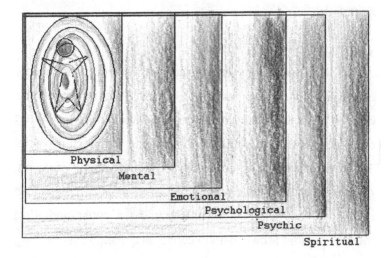

Figure 5:2 Energy bodies linked by the levels to time.

The twelve energy bodies all lie within the first level, that of the physical. Yet, all energy bodies connect to all levels at all times. The chakras are points at which energy bodies connect to energy levels. These levels are created by the interaction between the physical body and linear time. The energy bodies link the spirit to the physical realm. The levels link the physical realm to time. It is this link to time that is important when studying homeopathy. Because an event is located both in space and time, it is the interaction between these two realms that help to determine the homeopathic potency needed. **The energy body determines the remedy, and the level determines the potency. If the event occurred without the presence of time, no consideration of potency would be necessary.**

• Time

No event takes place in isolation. Without time, events occur but exist without meaning. It is possible for a person to be born without a link to time. A person born without a link to time will experience life as a series of unrelated and unconnected events. These events seem to occur randomly and without meaning. Actions exist but are disconnected from their consequences preventing the person from ever forming a cause-and-effect relationship that allows them to control their life.

It is also possible for a person to experience time differently on each of the levels. This person may appear overly wise for their years, or strikingly naive. A person experiencing time at a different rate from those around them always seems out of sync and is often viewed by others as mentally retarded, slow, gifted, astute, spiritual, blessed, or otherwise "different".

In Western scientific thought, time has always been viewed as a measurable constant. However, in the reality of the energy realms, time is a pliable, fluid, changeable medium that interacts with the physical realm to create the various levels that form what we call the personality. Higher potency remedies act upon these upper realms and alter their function while leaving the physical structure of the person unchanged. Lower potencies act upon the physical realm leaving the mental and emotional aspects of the person unchanged; unless the physical problems are impacting the mental state. **It is for this reason higher potencies are used mainly for mental and emotional aspects of the person while lower potencies are used mainly for physical aspects**. An exception to this general use of remedies is the use of high potencies administered immediately to stop problems from penetrating the energy bodies; as in sudden impact injuries or skin burns.

• Physical Events Become Emotional Problems

Any event which occurs in the physical realm will move throughout the various levels with time. For example, a car accident can result in physical trauma to the body. The physical trauma will penetrate from the outer energy bodies to the inner energy bodies quickly. If left untreated, it will begin moving through and manifesting in the various levels. Very shortly after the accident the person may find himself thinking continuously about the accident as it penetrates into the mental level. This is followed by a fear of driving or anxiety when thinking about the car accident or the injuries sustained as the trauma begins to penetrate the emotional level. Anxiety attacks and an inability to drive or ride in cars may become present as the trauma penetrates the psychological level. A foreboding or sense of doom when thinking about a car, or a belief that riding in the car may cause death, is often a manifestation of the trauma as it penetrates the psychic level. When the trauma has fully penetrated all the levels and has entered the spiritual level, a person may feel punished by God, haunted by demons or suffering karmic consequences.

It is important to understand that each and every event, both good and bad, that occurs in a person's life will move through all levels with time. Because of this, it is extremely important that bad events such as trauma or emotional upset be treated as quickly as possible to prevent their penetration into upper levels. If a person were to clear the bad events from the energy levels continuously throughout a lifetime, that person may end their life with a feeling of being blessed rather than persecuted.

Conventional medical science tends to view any manifestation above the physical level as a mental or emotional problem. No consideration is ever given to correcting the physical problem which has moved to and is now manifesting on the upper level. Allopathic medicine tends to divide the world into a strictly binary world of physical or mental. Because of this approach, psychiatrists and therapists have often spent years attempting to talk to or analyze a person in order to correct the problem. Unfortunately, because the original trauma and resulting problems still exist in the physical level, the "emotional" problems continued to occur. This misunderstanding of the actual situation has led to the current trend of placing patients on medication to cover over emotional symptoms and control behavior rather than to discover the underlying cause.

With a clear understanding of these concepts, the question of how homeopathy treats disturbances in the energy bodies and energy levels can now be answered. In order for a remedy to treat the energy bodies, it must first be converted from the physical realm into the energetic realm through a process known as potentization. **Only a potentized substance has the ability to make changes on the energy realm controlled by the affected energy body and, subsequently, on the physical body.**

6

Remedy Potentization

Samuel Hahnemann discovered that remedies could be made safe by diluting substances that could have been harmful or fatal if used in their pure material form. By diluting and potentizing his remedies, he found this new form worked even better for healing. He continued to dilute and potentize the amount of substance, until the remedies were reduced to only energy, where nothing material remained, and existed not in the realm of matter any longer, but in the realm of energy. It is this energetic medicine, working on an energy level that can create healing in the energy bodies of the individual who is sick.

In **Organon of Medicine**, paragraph 16, Hahnemann states:

> Our vital force, as a spirit-like dynamis, cannot be attacked and infected by injurious influences

on the healthy organism caused by the external inimical forces that disturb the harmonious play of life otherwise than in a spirit-like (dynamic) way, and in like manner all such morbid derangement's (disease) cannot be removed from it by the physician in any other way than by the spirit-like alternative powers of the serviceable medicines acting upon our spirit-like vital force, which preserves them through the medium of the sentient faculty of the nerves everywhere present in the organism, so that it is only by their dynamic action of the vital force that remedies are able to re-establish and do actually re-establish health and vital harmony after the changes in the health of the patient cognizable by our senses (the totality of the symptoms) have revealed the disease to the carefully observing and investigating physician as fully as was requisite in order to enable him to cure it.

In other words, since illness only occurs when our vital energy, our energy bodies, breakdown and allow it to occur, illness can only be relieved by a form of medicine that is also prepared to act in an energetic fashion.

• Potentizing Remedies

The process of potentizing starts with a dilution of any

remedy substance in a mixture of 10% substance to 90% medium. The medium would consist of whatever the remedy substance would dissolve into best, such as alcohol, water and alcohol, or lactose. This dilution is placed in a small vial. This mixture is shaken or succussed vigorously until completely blended. This new blended substance is again diluted to a mixture of 10% substance to 90% ratio of the medium in a second vial and again shaken. Ten percent of this newer shaken substance is diluted yet again with another 90% ratio of medium in a third vial and again shaken. The resulting mixture is a 3X homeopathic potency.

This process of diluting the resulting substance to the same ratio of medium is continued to further and further mixtures. At the point of reaching the twenty-fourth vial of blended and shaken mixtures, there are no molecules of the original substance detectable by measurement devices now available. However, the energy inherent in the original substance molecule has been expanded and is carried by the medium. Each dilution, by way of the blending of new medium and shaking process, has expanded and enhanced the presence of energy to a level greater than existed in each previous bottle.

The further the remedy has been diluted and succussed away from the original substance, the more powerful it is for healing. This may be difficult to understand in our present

day frame of mind where more is usually better, but it is--
nevertheless--the way it is--the way it has always been. This
principle will be clarified as the discipline of Quantum Physics
develops.

• More is Not Always Better

The idea that more is better applies only in the physical
realm--and there only in specific and limited instances. Although
a small amount of a vitamin may be useful, excessive amounts
of this same vitamin may be fatal because the amount of vital
force energy needed to store and convert it to a useful form may
deplete the body's vital force reserves.

Homeopathic medicine does not over tax the body in this
fashion for a very simple reason. The body must convert a material
substance into energy in order for it to be used. Sometimes the
energy necessary for the conversion is more than the body has
available. A homeopathic remedy is already reduced to energy,
using none of the body's vital force energy to convert it. The
homeopathic remedy is not only readily available, but actually
serves to reinforce and enhance the body's vital force.

• Substance Converted to Energy

In the process of potentization, a material substance
is transformed into energy. This process has been the basis of
disagreement between the allopathic (conventional medical)

community and the homeopathic community since the beginning. Allopathy doesn't recognize the existence of energy bodies, nor does it accept the concept of an energy signature affecting energy bodies. Allopathy views the body as a chemical component which can only be affected by the addition of other chemicals. The reliance on the energetic signatures of substances vs. their chemical composition has been the basis of the argument to discredit homeopathy--nothing material remains in a potentized remedy, and therefore, in a chemically based system it can do nothing. How each new potency becomes more powerful than the last when there is nothing in the remedy is the question that remains.

• More Powerful with Each Dilution

Molecules are composed of atoms in specific arrangements and concentrations. As scientists have finally discovered, atoms--the basic building blocks of all matter--are actually particles of solidified energy which are arranged in specific energy fields and have unique energetic signatures. These molecules can combine with other molecules to form various substances known as compounds--each with its unique energetic signature. It is the uniqueness of this energetic signature that accounts for the ability of the substance to interact in energy fields and bring about specific changes in those fields.

When energy is added into a molecule or compound, the energy field of that molecule or compound is expanded while keeping its unique arrangement and energetic signature. In order for this expansion to take place, a neutral medium, which can be absorbed into the molecular energy pattern, must surround the molecule to allow the original molecule's energetic signature to expand without hindrance. This is the basic concept behind the process known as potentization.

• Energy Expands

Let's start at the beginning. When a substance, even an inert one like sand (pure silica sand is ground with lactose until it is soluble in liquid) is placed in a bottle at a dilution of 10% to 90% of the neutral medium, alcohol or lactose, and succussed (shaken violently against a hard object twenty times) the energetic signature inherent to the substance is released and expands as it absorbs the medium. After all the medium has been absorbed by the expanding energy, further shaking will have no additional effect on the strength of the remedy as it cannot expand further until new medium is added. This first product is known as a 1X potency. Each time the material is prepared in this fashion, it is known as a potentized substance, commonly called a potency.

In the second dilution, 10% of the first bottle is placed in a bottle with 90% more alcohol. Again the mixture is shaken twenty times. As the new medium is added and absorbed, the energy signature of the original molecule continues to expand until all of the newly added medium has been absorbed. As this process is repeated in the next bottle, the same thing occurs. The energy signature from the previous bottle will expand by absorbing the new medium when shaken. The second product is known as a 2X potency.

This process can be repeated again and again. Each time new medium is added, the energy signature can expand even more. As the energy signature expands, it becomes larger and more powerful than it was in any of the previous potencies. Each time the material is potentized, the number before the X is increased by one, indicating the number of times the material has been processed. The X in this case represents the dilution of 10% to 90% on the decimal scale.

It is very important to understand that it is not the process of diluting the material, nor is it simply the action of shaking the material which increases its strength. The strength of the homeopathic material is enhanced by the interaction between these two events. A substance is placed in a neutral medium which can be absorbed into the original energy signature, thereby, allowing that signature to expand. The process of shaking the material causes this absorption to take place. Neither of these actions in and of itself, performed alone, has any effect on the strength of the potentized remedy.

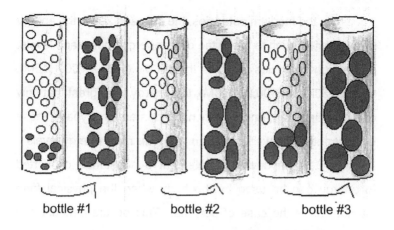

bottle #1   bottle #2   bottle #3

A substance is put in a bottle with alcohol as a medium and shaken. The energy signature of each molecule gets larger each time new medium is added and the bottle is shaken. The energy signature of the molecules will fill all the available space in the medium.

Figure 6:1 Shaking expands energy to fill the entire bottle.

In the lower potencies, the 3's, 6's and 9's, there are still a few molecules present, but these are insignificant if one is looking from a chemical viewpoint. However, the energy of the molecules has expanded enough to make these potencies cause some reaction in the body of a patient who takes it. This reaction is mainly in the lower energy bodies inside the physical body. A low potency will convert upward, eventually reaching higher energy bodies, but never downward to lower energy bodies.

In the medium potencies, the 30's and 200's, the energy is powerful enough to get to the outer energy bodies and levels. In the high potencies, such as the 1000's (1M), 10,000 (10M), 50,000 (50M), or 100,000 (CM), the energy is so great that only one dose is taken, and usually not repeated for a year. These highest potencies work mainly in the outer most energy levels.

It is important to note that a substance converted to energy can be used by the body when the physical form cannot—as is the case of poisons. This occurs because the amount of vital force needed to convert the material substance to an energetic form exceeds the body's vital energy capacities or capabilities (the poisonous substance exhausts the vital force). Because a homeopathic substance is not in its chemical form, it cannot affect the body on a chemical level. A person cannot be poisoned by a homeopathically prepared substance even if that substance is chemically poisonous in a material form.

Substances which are chemically inert or unavailable for use by the body in their original material form will work in a homeopathic form. An excellent example is the substance commonly called sand. Pure silica sand is the substance plants use to hold up against the wind. A person who is low in silica has trouble standing up to the pressures and winds of change in life. By taking homeopathically potentized silica, Silicea in Latin, the problem is corrected. This substance would do nothing for the individual who digested it in its pure non-homeopathic forms.

• Potentized Energy Becomes a Remedy

The molecular pattern of a substance becomes an energy pattern that can be used to adjust and modify the individual's energy fields. Based on the rule of "like cures like", a substance that will cause certain symptoms will cure the same symptoms in a person who displays those symptoms--matching energy for energy, the energy of the potentized homeopathic remedy to the energy body and level of the sick individual.

• The Difference Between C's and X's

There are two forms of homeopathic remedies, X and C potencies. In the potentizing process, if the first bottle is 10% of the substance and 90% of the medium, the potency is an X, indicating the Roman Numeral 10. In the potentizing process, if the first bottle is 1% of the substance and 99% of the medium, the potency is a C, indicating the Roman Numeral 100.

The distinction seems to create a state of confusion among homeopathic practitioners. Many do not fully understand the difference between the chemical world and the energetic world.

Energy has a nature and character distinct from matter. One cannot take a principle that applies to matter and apply it to the energy form and expect it to be correct. This confusion has led to disagreement among the various schools of homeopathy.

Without a clear understanding of the conceptual basis upon which homeopathic principles rest, certain individuals have made judgments about energy based on their knowledge of matter. The deductions are incorrect and misleading and have led to some seriously flawed teachings.

As a substance is diluted into the energy of a potency, the number of times the medium is changed and the energy expanded further is what is important. In other words, the potency number, the 6, 12, 30 or 200 determines the relative strength of the potentized remedy, not the dilution strength of the original substance.

An example of this error in thinking can be illustrated by comparing two stacks of paper, each with 30 sheets. One stack consisting of paper sheets 8 inches by 11 inches in size, and the other stack of paper sheets 11 inches by 14 inches in size. If the paper is the same grade, the two stacks will be of equal height regardless of their length and width. When dealing with the energy of a homeopathically prepared potency, it is not how much one started with, but how many times it is succussed and allowed to expand into new medium that determines its strength. A 30th potency of an X may have started with more chemical substance, but after the 30th potentizing, it is identical in strength energetically to a 30th potency of a C, which started with less substance chemically.

8X11 inches   11X14 inches

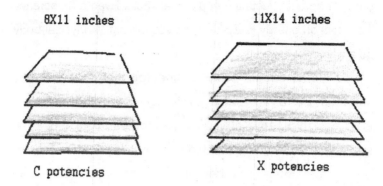

C potencies   X potencies

The same number of sheets in each stack of paper makes each stack the same height, no matter how large each sheet is.

Figure 6:2 The number of potencies is what matters, not the amount of substance.

This concept is true even in the lowest potencies where there may still be a few molecules of substance in measurable quantity. It is important to remember that homeopathic substances are not concerned with the chemical components from which they are derived. The expansion of energy is what makes a remedy a potency--not how big the material dose was originally.

A material dose of a chemical substance affects the body on the gross cellular level. As a substance is potentized, the effect moves from the individual cells to the various energy bodies where it affects the body as a whole. Even a 3x potency will affect an energy body that involves the entire physical body as a whole.

Some people have commented that an X potency still must be larger--since an 11 x14 inch sheet of paper is larger than an 8x11inch sheet of paper. Think of a substance in a vial as millions of little red balls, full of energy and potential. When the medium is added this may appear as little white balls, inert and non-reactive. As the vial is shaken, the white balls are absorbed into the red balls—expanding them. This takes place each time the medium is changed and the vial is shaken. The red balls become larger and larger until they have absorbed all of the white balls. There is no difference in how many of the red balls there were to begin with. They are all red and act in the same way--whether the original vial had 10% of the red balls to begin with, or only 1% --they are all going to act as if they are red balls after the vial is shaken.

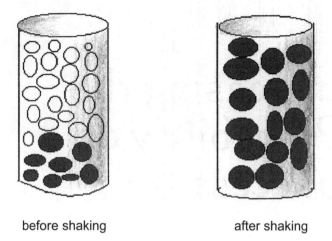

before shaking   after shaking

Figure 6:3 Energy expands into the medium until distinction
between substance and medium disappears.

The important thing to remember is that homeopathy works on energy levels and in no way resembles chemical medicine. The understanding of this reality opens the door for the use of homeopathic remedies in all treatment venues.

7

Increasing the Probability of Success

As with all healing modalities, no matter how skilled the practitioner, no matter how diligent the client, no matter how intense the efforts, there are times when a symptom or disease will not be relieved. Often the allopathic medical community will sight this as proof that homeopathic remedies do not work. Often the practitioner will feel this is due to lack of skill on their part and will continue to suggest remedy after remedy hoping for "the miracle". Often a client will desperately go from practitioner to practitioner and modality to modality desperately searching for the "source of healing". In each modality, the practitioner and client must recognize that there are limits to the healing ability of the body and that some incidents of failure will occur.

In homeopathic therapies, failure means that nothing happens. There are no toxic chemicals or undesirable side effects that could worsen the condition or weaken the health of the person. Although it is true that a person may allow a "curable" condition such as cancer to progress beyond its "curable" stage by avoiding standard allopathic treatment, this is a choice that each person has the freedom to make. It is important for the homeopathic practitioner to encourage a client to seek immediate evaluation by a licensed health care practitioner for any serious and potentially life-threatening condition. Homeopathy is not in conflict with allopathic medicine. This is an extremely important point to understand. Homeopathy can be used by the client simultaneously to ameliorate symptoms and provide support to conventional treatment.

In homeopathy, as with all other convention and non-conventional therapies, treatment will be successful 65-70% of the time. One third of all patients will not find relief and must seek help from other modalities. This is an actuality that can be confirmed by any doctor or alternative practitioner. However, a clear understanding of several homeopathic principles will enhance the likelihood of success when using remedies.

Even if all the rules and methods are followed, there will still be times when the potency or the remedy does not work. This can happen because a problem may appear to be physical when it is, in fact, emotional. It is also possible that what is first believed to be an emotional problem may instead be the manifestation of a physical problem left to penetrate to the upper levels. In each of these cases, no matter how carefully the remedy has been chosen, the clearing of the underlying problem does not completely take place. This is due to the misunderstanding of the source of the original problem. By carefully researching the symptoms, clearing each new symptom as it occurs after each administration of a remedy, and listening carefully to all aspects of the person's problems, it may be possible to ultimately reach the source of the original affliction.

It is also possible that the correct remedy has been chosen, but it has been given in an inappropriate potency. In the process of potentizing, each progressive potency expands the energy field of the substance as new medium is added. The molecules of energy get larger with each potency. The energy of the potency fills the appropriate energy body to the correct level. The potency has to be large enough to fill that level in order to push problems out and away from the physical body. When the structure of the energy body is complete, nothing can penetrate to cause disease, nor can the vital force leak out. **The right size potency of the correctly chosen remedy will make the energy body complete**.

• Understand Vital Force

It is important that the person seeking to use homeopathy as a healing modality has a clear understanding of the concepts of vital force and energy bodies. With this understanding, it is possible to recognize the reason why a remedy succeeded or the reason why it did not. In the event of "failure" of a remedy, this understanding can allow the practitioner to take the next logical step, thereby increasing the likelihood of success.

Vital force is the energy of life. As has been previously discussed, this concept has been recognized in all cultures throughout time. Without this vital force, life is not possible. The difference between the living body and the dead body is quite simply the presence of this vital force in the living body.

Where there is a break down in the energy body, the protective shield formed by that energy body is incomplete. This allows disease causing organisms to penetrate, creating what we recognize as illness within the person. These incomplete energy bodies can also result in malfunctions which allow problems, or permit the vital force to dissipate through the gaps in the incomplete energy bodies.

Often a person will say, "Nothing is wrong with me, really, but I feel so incomplete." Language can actually reflect what a person knows, on a subconscious level, about what is happening in the body.

• An Energy Body Sphere

Energy bodies are actually circles of solid bands of energy, shifted around the physical body to complete a sphere. Each body is a complete sphere with multiple parts that pivot around the head and the feet. Each individual person has a pattern of circles (grouplets) in these spheres that is different from any other individual, although there are common patterns among them. That is why one has to match the remedy to a pattern. The molecular pattern in the remedy has to match the circles shifted in the pattern of the energy body, the evidence of which is the symptom complex.

A single sphere may have a problem that is affecting only that sphere. When it is made solid again with the right potency of the right remedy, the sphere stops losing its vital force and the symptoms diminish. It is similar to an air-conditioned house. If the windows and doors are closed tight, the cold air does not leak out. The right potency is the one right for the energy level the sphere is working on. The right remedy is the one that matches the pattern of the circles of energy within the sphere.

If the disease is caught quickly, the energy body can be made solid and repair itself. That is why a single remedy can clear up all the symptoms. If the problem has gone on for a while and has moved into larger energy bodies affecting adjacent energy bands, many remedies over a period of time will be needed to clear the problem.

If the remedy is not correct, its energy will just refill an already full sphere and the individual feels as though nothing has happened.

These bands are in different positions in each individual—that is why a disease in one person will be totally different in another person and why several people with the same disease will manifest different symptoms. Everybody has the same bands, just in different patterns. If a practitioner tries to give the same constitutional remedy to everyone, in spite of different disease manifestations, the results will be limited and success will be achieved in only those few clients whose bands happen to match the remedy given.

• Remedies That Just Do What They Do

Some remedies do not need to be matched to individuals and can be given to anyone. There are two major remedies that act as glue to help the bands of all the energy bodies hold together. These are Arnica Montana for the physical aspects (injury) and Ignatia (Ignatia Amara) for the emotional aspects (grief). These remedies work on the whole person no matter where the trauma or grief originated, although the right potency to the right energy level works best. Arnica makes the bands hold together and stops the physical trauma. Ignatia does the same on emotional trauma. When in need of Ignatia, a person may actually comment that they feel as if they are falling apart.

There are only two glues, but there can be universal remedies that will work on grouplets of circles within spheres. This is because all human beings must share common characteristics reflected in the arrangement of the bands. For example, all people share common bands which govern the nervous and digestive systems. Hypericum for pain and Ipecacuanha for vomiting are two universal remedies that work the same way on every person because of the common grouplets all people share.

• Think of an Orchestra

The example of an orchestra may illustrate the difference between the actions of remedies given for different problems. The constitutional remedy that affects the whole person and changes things in every part of the body--which must be matched to the individual--would be the example of the entire orchestra playing the symphony. There may be one person in each section having a problem with the music of the piece being played.

A second example would be that of one section, for instance the violins. This would be likened to a system in the body that is having problems, such as the digestive tract, the respiratory system, or hormones being out of balance. Many remedies are known to have an affiliation with one particular system, such as Antimonium Tart. for the respiratory system, or Sepia for female hormonal problems.

A third example would be one instrument that is not being played correctly. This can be likened to one organ being affected, such as the eyes, the throat, the liver or the kidneys. A common example of this concept would be Euphrasia, which is most often the remedy for any eye affliction.

A fourth example would be the conductor rewriting the music that will affect the overall sound of the symphony. This can be likened to the mental enhancement remedies that rewrite everything in the central nervous system. Natrum Mur. in a high potency for improving information processing is a good example.

The fifth example would be the universal sound of the drums which are used in nearly every orchestra and nearly every piece of music worldwide. This can be likened to the remedies that just do what is expected of them, such as Arnica, Ignatia, Hypericum for nerve pain and Ipecacuanha to stop the symptom of vomiting.

• Some Problems Can't be Changed

Grouplets are patterns of placement of circles that govern various functions of the organism. If all the circles in a grouplet are positioned correctly, everything is functional, such as the grouplet for fertility. If there is an infertility problem, it could be that something in the grouplet is misplaced, not connected or lacking complete energy. If the problem is an incomplete band or grouplet that is not fully connected to the energy body, the right remedy could correct the problem. However, if something is not correct in the grouplet or is missing entirely, and it has always been this way, as in congenital problems, no potency or remedy can work. No remedy can restore something that was never there.

When grouplets are broken or sections are misplaced away from the grouplet, major problems of function in the organism cannot be fixed. The person will not be able to get rid of all the symptoms related to the problem no matter how well intentioned the practitioner. In these cases, the practitioner will find a point where many of the symptoms have been alleviated but the basic underlying problem still remains. Patients and practitioners must realize there are times when nothing more can be done and it is no one's fault. Not every problem can be completely fixed. That is just the way it is.

In these rare cases, homeopathy still offers benefits in its ability to support the person and prevent the problem from progressing and causing dysfunction is other areas. For example, an inability to conceive may be a dysfunctional problem that cannot be solved. This may lead to depression or feelings of worthlessness which can be corrected by remedies to help the individual live a fully functional life.

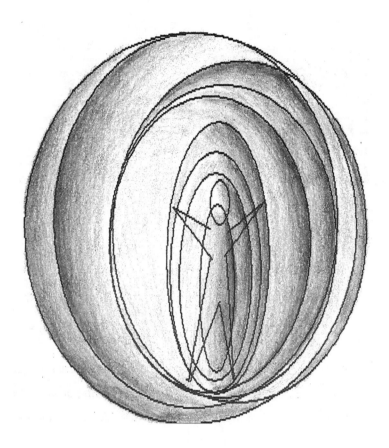

Grouplets are patterns of placement of circles that form a sphere around the body.

Figure 7:1   An energy body forms a complete sphere.

8

Potency Interaction on Energy Bodies and Levels

A total of twelve spherical energy bodies surround and animate the physical body of each living individual. The energy bodies form to link the pure energy of the soul to the material workings of the physical body. Without the presence of energy bodies, the soul would not be able to inhabit or animate the flesh and blood of the living body. Babies developing in the womb pattern the first four energy bodies after the birth mother. This is why adoption is always a difficult transition in spite of our best intensions.

Six more energy bodies are formed while the child grows, learns and develops through life. The remaining two develop at the end of life as the individual prepares to exit the material substance of the body and return to a pure energy existence.

The twelve energy bodies all lie within the first level, that of the physical. These levels are created by the interaction between the physical body and linear time. The energy bodies link the spirit to the physical realm. The levels link the physical realm to time. It is this link to time that is important when studying homeopathy. Because an event is located both in space and time, it is the interaction between these two realms that help to determine the homeopathic potency needed.

• Trauma's Effects

A trauma that occurs from a physical injury will first impact the outer energy bodies and penetrate inward, deeper and deeper through time. The inward penetration can be stopped by a high potency of a homeopathic remedy for trauma, such as Arnica Montana. Arnica taken in a 200 or 1000 potency as soon as possible after an injury occurs will help arrest the time duration of the trauma and help the body come back to normal. In many cases, the best results would be achieved by frequent doses of this higher potency for a period of a few hours after the traumatic event.

That is to say, doses of Arnica Montana in a 200 or 1M potency can be given every ten minutes for a period of two hours after a trauma has occurred. When this regime is used, it is not unusual for the trauma to have little or no lasting physical effect.

The use of a high potency after trauma must be immediate, for after a bit of time, and after the trauma has become an established physical injury or problem, a lower potency, such as a 6, 9 or 12 is more appropriate in order to push the problem out from deep inside the energy bodies.

A low potency given over a month's time is appropriate if the trauma is very old in order to clear it from the inside energy bodies and all of the energy levels.

Have you ever had a severe bump to the head? In the first few hours it hurts a lot and may feel hot, but there is no bruising or swelling. After a short time, swelling begins as blood and fluids start to seep into the tissues. The next day, the site of the injury is quite swollen and appears black and blue. As time progresses, the area continues to become more bruised. Three or four days later, the area is very tender, and the accumulated blood has seeped down to other parts of the face while turning a variety of colors. After this occurs, it takes weeks to get back to normal.

If a high potency of Arnica is taken right away, at the time the injury occurs, much of the bruising will not happen, since the injury would have been slowed or stopped in the outer energy bodies and kept from penetrating inward to do damage over time. At the same time the Arnica can prevent the injury from moving into the higher levels and manifesting as mentally based problems such as fear of falling or fear of other types of accidents.

• Viral Protection

This style of dosing is also effective for the onset of an acute viral infection. If a person were to take a high potency, a 200 or 1M, of the right remedy just as they are beginning to feel ill, the potency could stop the progress of the illness as it penetrates in from the outer energy bodies to the inner energy bodies. This works best when taken as the person just feels off, just beginning to feel sick with no actual symptoms other than feeling tired, or loss of appetite, or as headache and sore throat just begin to appear. Aconitum Nap. (Aconite) in a 200th potency, taken three times in one hour—3 doses, 30 minutes apart—is very effective. I have seen this course of action stop the flu completely by the time the last dose is taken.

If the symptom of a sore throat or fever is already present and progressing to more complex symptoms, a 30th potency of Aconitum taken every ten minutes for two hours is more appropriate to stop the progress of a flu or cold.

• Emotional Trauma

If the trauma is of an emotional nature, such a sudden grief, the same principles would apply. In this case, the immediate remedy would be Ignatia (Ignatia Amara) in a 200 or 1000 potency (1M), taking one dose or three doses in a 12 hour period. By using this remedy at the time of grief, it is possible to help stop the emotional trauma from entering the lower energy bodies and becoming a problem on the physical level. If left untreated, the initial emotional trauma will ultimately move into the upper levels where it could manifest itself as a different problem such as paranoia or depression.

In my practice I have seen many people who were affected by grief that was untreated and had penetrated inward, becoming a physical illness. I remember one young man who came to me with a sinus infection. During the interview, I asked him how long he had been suffering from this infection. He thought for a moment, then commented; "Oh, probably since the funeral." A single potency of Ignatia 200 cleared this problem even though it had already become physical. A single 200th potency dose of Ignatia worked because it had started in the spiritual realm of the outer levels.

It is appropriate with emotional trauma to use a high potency--even though the trauma has become physical--because the emotional, psychological and psychic level problems require a different approach. These problems began in the outer levels and, therefore, require higher potencies.

If a person takes a 1000 potency of Ignatia at the time of the grief, the physical problems will not occur. Although, any potency of Ignatia at any time after a grief situation will be helpful, the most effective dose would the 1M as soon as possible.

Ignatia is an amazing remedy for emotional grief in

helping the body to handle the problem. Think of how often you have seen a grief stricken person become unable to sleep or eat, start to lose weight and begin to look run down or become unable to focus on anything else. After the use of Ignatia 30 taken three times a day for three days any time after grief, the person can carry on with normal life. The grief is not forgotten, just handled by the body in the appropriate way.

If a grief problem has existed for a very long time, since childhood or adolescence, it could have become a deep-seated physical problem. In this case, Ignatia 6X given over a period of a month can work to clear the problem from deep in the energy bodies in the physical level.

It is a good idea for all of us to take Iqnatia 6X for the duration of a month at some time in our adult life. This is because most, if not all of us have grief, shame and fear that originated in childhood experiences that we have forgotten. It is common to go on in life thinking these little emotional traumas of the past have no effect, when in reality, they have affected us greatly. Be warned, taking Ignatia in a 6X will bring many of these traumas into the mind as they clear out of the physical level. It is important in this therapy not to stop taking the remedy until the month has been completed. When the memories surface, the individual is prone to the same feeling as when the trauma occurred, leaving the person feeling retched and angry. If the person stops using the Ignatia, the feelings take a while to clear. If the person takes an extra dose if Ignatia 6X (up to 5 doses in a 24 hour period are okay) and continues the remedy for the duration of the month, the feelings clear soon after taking the extra dose. At the end of the month, it is not unusual for the person to comment on new feelings of joy--with a renewed calmness in their life.

Another remedy that addresses emotional upset is Natrum Muriaticum. The person in need of Ignatia will deny they have a problem and may wish to be alone and unaided in their grief. The person in need of Natrum Mur. will say something similar to the idea that they were happy before, but now they are always sad and can not function. The brain needs sodium chloride to carry out the function of placing events into the proper filing system and out of the active mind. Not surprisingly, a person in this situation will begin to crave salt where there was no craving before. By taking Natrum Mur.(the potentized form of sodium chloride), the brain gets the chemical it needs to function. The craving will ease and the person will feel a resolve in the grief situation.

I saw a client once who had been angry at her mother for many years but did not know why. She took Natrum Mur. for another problem. During the process she relived a drowning experience where she had become angry with her mother for not noticing she was in danger. Her anger dissipated at that time.

• Biochemical Problems

Illness that is due to biochemical imbalances and auto-immune problems will begin in the middle energy bodies that occur just inside the physical body and penetrate outward. These are usually due to an accumulation of emotional baggage one carries through life that interrupts energy flow and normal function. If this is the case, a mid-level (30th) potency of a remedy that matches the symptoms of the person overall can be used to push the problem out and allow the body to heal. This is the situation where multiple problems get compacted together and many remedies are needed to clear the layers of life's accumulation of dilemmas. These are the most frequent cases that a practitioner would see in a homeopathic practice. It is suitable to start with a well chosen remedy in a 30th potency. If the problem returns after a period of amelioration, but in a slightly different form, move to the 200th potency. If the first symptom is relieved, but a totally new symptom becomes dominant, use a complement of the first remedy in a 30th potency, working symptom by symptom, carefully monitoring changes, until all the symptoms are gone and the person is clear and well.

If the first symptoms come back and the same remedy given in higher potencies does not help, the problem was not what it seemed and the practitioner needs to look at it in a different way and use an entirely different approach and remedy.

I once saw a client with a swelling in the prostate gland that restricted the flow of urine. He tried all the common remedies for the prostate and urinary tract problems such as Digitalis, Berberis Vul., Cantharis and Staphysagria. Nothing helped. After looking at the problem not as a prostate problem but as a problem of swelling due to heavy metal accumulation in glandular tissue through lifestyle toxicity, we were able to drain the heavy metals using Phosphorus 30, followed by chord potencies of Zincum Met. and Alumina (a remedy made from aluminum, possibly from soda cans). (chord potencies are described in Chapter 9) What ultimately worked in this situation was looking at the problem from a different point of view instead of giving up.

• Skin Problems

Problems that manifest as skin trouble such as rashes, eczema, or psoriasis are only symptoms of deeper problems. When a mid-level, 15th or 30th, potency of a remedy that matches the person is taken, the problem will be pushed from the inner energy bodies to the outside and out of the individual. As the problem passes the energy body that corresponds to the skin, the rash will aggravate, giving the patient a few hours or days of discomfort. As the problem pushes out of all the energy bodies, the skin symptom will disappear and the individual will be relieved of the problem—the skin problem as well as the underlying cause.

I once treated a person with what appeared to be a slight case of eczema between her fingers. She also complained of depression and sleep problems. I carefully studied her case and she took a remedy that I considered a good match to her symptoms. In just a few days her hands became raw with oozing open sores. She was very uncomfortable for a couple of weeks, but the amazing thing was that her depression disappeared, her sleep improved, and I could see a definite clearing in her entire body. Her posture improved, her eyes sparkled, and her spirit lightened. It was amazing to see. Even though she had to endure a difficult situation for a time, the benefits were well worth the effort. This was an unusually severe case and I have never before seen such an aggravation, but it is a good example of the powerful effect homeopathy can achieve.

• Using Too High a Potency

There are some homeopathic practitioners who use very high potencies, 10,000, 50,000th and 100,000th attenuations as constitutional remedies. The problem with the use of such high potencies for chronic problems is that they only work in the outer psychic and spiritual energy levels, and therefore, will work only on spiritually and psychically based problems. Potencies this high may create a temporary amelioration of physical problems, but it will only be temporary. Instead of realizing the limitation of the high potency approach, many insist that outside factors must have worked to counteract the action of the remedies, rendering them useless. In an attempt to thwart or anticipate this problem, many practitioners insist their clients follow austere regimes while being treated—never realizing the remedy is only skirting the outer energy bodies and changes nothing in the lower energy bodies where the problems originate. Repetition of these high doses does nothing more than cause the remedy to antidote itself, rendering it ineffective.

A remedy given in the high potency of 10,000 (10M) for mental enhancement purposes and in the 1,000 (1M) to solve spiritual and psychic based problems will be effective and permanent in action. In these cases, the remedy is given in one dose, and not repeated again for a least a year.

The high potencies of 50,000 and 100,000 (CM) are so high as to have no correlation to any energy body. Even when given for mental enhancement, these remedies may produce only temporary results.

• Review

To review, potencies of 30 are best used for problems of constitutional origin, such as those present from birth and carried forth from past generations in the physical inheritance of the body or the past life experiences of the soul. These can manifest as biochemical imbalances, mineral absorption problems or as skin problems, but will affect the entire body at once.

Potencies of 200 or 1000 (1M) are best used for immediate trauma, both physical and emotional, to stop the penetration of the trauma from outside inward toward the physical body.

Potencies of 6X clear emotional and physical trauma from the long ago past, as far back as childhood, and can also be used for the absorption of minerals missing in the cells of the body.

Potencies of 10,000 (10M) are best used to enhance the function of the intellect and mental power. Single doses of the 1,000 (1M) potency can correct a malfunction in mental processing.

Potencies of 50,000 (50M) or 100,000 (CM) do not have an energy body equivalent and will only create temporary results.

Remedies diluted on scales of X or C work in the same manner. When purchasing remedies, no care need be taken in whether a remedy is an X or a C potency.

This is how remedies work best, providing consistent results--by impacting the energy body and level affected with the potentized-energy-converted substance that best matches the problem.

• No Need to Abstain

The good news is that when following this model for

the use of potency, there is no need to abstain from all of the substances prohibited in the practices of the past. In other words, when taking a homeopathic remedy, it is okay to drink coffee, mint tea, chocolate and milk. There is no need to stay away from menthol, eucalyptus, camphor or mint. It is okay to use caffeine, alcoholic beverages and cigarette smoke. Although there are other very good reasons to abstain or limit these substances, they will not interfere with the use of homeopathic remedies.

The reason these are no longer prohibited is clear in the reality of the energy model of homeopathy. A potentized remedy is converted to energy and cannot be interfered with by a material substance that stays in the physical body and does not enter the energy bodies. If a remedy does not work or stops working too soon, it did not come in contact with an antidote substance, but rather was not chosen correctly in potency to begin with.

9

Combinations VS. Single Remedies

Through the years, various individuals have attempted to simplify the process of choosing the right remedy and potency for each individual. Many have designed various memory schemes that will allow the practitioner to know which remedies to recommend for each disease. Others have attempted to discover some "magic" formula by which the strength of each potency can be calculated so that the exact strength needed can be determined. Most have recognized that it is not possible to keep all the information that is necessary to make the proper choice of the correct remedy and potency for each individual in the front of one's mind. To help streamline the problem, various forms of combinations have been developed.

Some combinations were created by combining multiple remedies into a single preparation. If there are five remedies that are known to be helpful for migraine headaches, all five are combined into a single product and sold for migraine headaches. People can buy these combinations anytime without the advice or help of anyone. There are many combinations on the market that can be useful for short term acute illness and symptoms that are self-limiting even without treatment. These combinations can help the person feel better by getting rid of their symptoms fast--often bringing relief that is not possible from over-the-counter chemically-based products.

Combination remedies can be a good choice for the immediate relief of very simple problems. In cases where a homeopathic practitioner is not readily available, these combinations do allow the uninformed novice to select a homeopathic preparation based on a very simple understanding of the package instructions. These preparations can allow a person to discover some of the many benefits possible with homeopathic treatments. Their safety makes these remedies, in most cases, preferable over chemically-based products which can have unintended side effects. Every product that has been developed for use in the homeopathic field over the years has a time and a place where it is applicable, but it is necessary to understand when a product is appropriate.

• Not for Long Term Use

Combinations are not meant for long term use or chronic problems. Combinations will not change biochemistry to bring about lasting relief from chronic problems. The reason for this limitation lies in the way the remedies are put together in these combinations and interact with each other. It is possible to create a false platform where only a limited amount of healing action can be expected. This is particularly true when attempting to use a combination for a chronic problem. It may appear at first that the symptoms are going away and the combination is working, but the effect does not last. It is similar to building a step put together with several planks of wood that are not actually attached. If a person were to take a step onto those planks, the plank step would collapse and fall apart. The action of the combination remedy will collapse and fall away with any amount of stress the person experiences, just as the false step would.

• Homeopathic Chords

Some combinations are multiple potencies of the same remedy. These multiple potency combinations are known as chords. These preparations contain a single remedy such as Calcarea Carb. However, instead of a single potency level, the preparation may contain multiple potencies that have been placed into the same globule. A typical chord of Calcarea Carb.

may contain potencies of 3C, 12C, 30C, and 60C all together in one globule.

At the time these chord remedies were developed, it was believed these potencies would remain separate and would not blend into one large potency, or perhaps average themselves out to a mid-range level. Many homeopaths who lacked a full and complete understanding of how to select the different potencies, believed that the use of these combinations could simplify the process of choosing potency because the right potency would be selected by the body and the others would simply "vanish".

According to one theory, if it is difficult to choose a potency that is correct, many potencies in one remedy can provide the correct potency, and the vibration level of each individual patient would take only the potency needed.

Another theory touts ease of administration. Changing the potency during the course of an illness is unnecessary since the resonating potency would correctly match the disease as it changes vibration levels in its course of action. Still another theory is that the body can average the chords together to create a potency not found in the original combination. For example, in the Calcarea Carb. chord the body could average the 3C and the 12C to create a 7C potency. It was also believed that the body could create any potency needed simply by adding together the full range of the potencies in the chord. In the example of Calcarea Carb., the body would be able to create any potency from 3C to I05C based on its ability to add these potencies together. Unfortunately, all of these theories were based on a chemical model that is not fully applicable in homeopathy.

These chords were first described in the early twentieth century by Dr. Cahis of Barcelona. He was the first to prepare and use single remedies in multiple potencies. He likened such preparations to musical melodies, or chords, and discovered that the therapeutic action of the multiple potencies worked differently than single potencies. It wasn't until the 1970's that the application of these remedies became widespread and the variety of theories concerning their use became apparent.

• Not the Way it Seems

The problem with these theories is that energy has its own properties and does not obey chemical laws. In chemistry, all compounds that are added together have a cumulative and interacting effect, while in energy each signature remains distinct and unique and, therefore, cannot be used to create this cumulative effect. Because of this unique property of energy, the combination of potencies does not always do what it is predicted to do.

In the energetic model, it is the energy of the lower potencies that rule over the higher potencies because the lower potencies are "heavier". The higher potencies, because of their "lighter weight", move more quickly and establish themselves in the upper energy fields prior to the action of the lower potencies. When the lower potencies are combined with the higher potencies, the lower ones fall through the platforms created by the higher potencies leaving a hole through which all lower potencies fall. Because of this property, all but the lowest potency drains out of the body. Not only is there none of the higher potencies left to work, but these "holes" can actually drain out a previous single remedy that was helping. If there is any curative effect from the chord, it will be found in the lowest potency of the chord, which will remain after all higher potencies have drained--since the lowest potency rules over all others. The therapeutic effect would be from the lowest potency, the 3C is the only one actually being utilized.

There are times when a multiple potency and the drainage effect is desirable, such as with Zinc, but it is important that one be aware of what is really happening. The use of a multiple potency chord of Natrum Muriaticum could be very helpful in draining excess accumulations of salt from the body. A chord of Alumina could be useful for draining excess aluminum accumulated from drinking soda from cans when that action is needed, but chords are not appropriate when a remedy needs to remain in the body.

• When Not to Use a Chord

A friend of mine once suffered a severe head trauma in a serious car accident. For years after she used calcium antacids constantly. She explained that the calcium in the antacids controlled the seizures she was prone to. There was a constant acidity in her stomach in response to the use of the antacids. I suggested the possibility of using Calcarea Carb. as a homeopathic form of calcium that would be more readily absorbed by the cells that needed the calcium, thus relieving her need to constantly renew a source of calcium. She was willing to try.

After her first course of treatment with Calcarea Carb. in a 30th potency taken three times a day for three days, she noticed that the acidity in her stomach was gone and she stopped taking the antacids. She was also completely free of seizures. She was antacid free and seizure free for several months.

Some time later she tried a new product being marketed by a new company. It was Calcarea Carb. in a multiple chord potency with 3C, 12C, 30C, 60C all together in the same remedy. She reported that all the good effects she had received from homeopathic calcium had been wiped out by this product. She experienced the return of the stomach acidity and several seizures over a short period of time, but reported that they never reached the previous level of intensity she had experienced prior to her first homeopathic remedy. The calcium that had been put in place by the single remedy was drained by the chord.

• The Drainage Effect

Homeopathic potencies, when given one at a time, arrange themselves on top of each other, similar to a stack of layers on a cake. Because the lower potencies are "heavier", they move into place at a slower speed and must be allowed to settle into place before the next lighter, faster potency is added. In multiple potency combinations, the top layers move into place faster than the heavier lower layers. This arrangement is much like placing the smaller layers onto the cake plate before adding the larger layers, which results in an unstable structure that will collapse the entire cake. To keep potencies in the body, they must be built up from lower to higher attenuations, just as a cake--the lighter layers on top of the heavier ones.

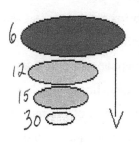 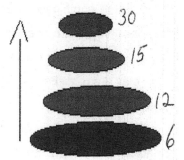

Lower potencies
are heavier and
will collapse onto
higher potencies

Higher potencies
used after lower
potencies build upon
a solid foundation

Figure 9:1 Lower potencies collapse through lighter,
higher potencies and drain out of the body.
Using lower potencies first and building to
higher potencies creates the right foundation.

• Substance Overload

There are times when a problem is caused by an
overload of a certain substance. Even a nutrient that is needed
can occur in overload if consumed in excessive amounts or over
a prolonged period of time. In a case of overload, a chord of the
offending substance will help drain it from the body. The lowest
potency that remains helps the body resolve its problems with
absorption or detoxification, depending whether the substance
is essential or harmful.

Some combinations are multiple remedies in multiple potencies. These are used for draining toxic substances from the body. Like any other combination, there is a time and a place where they are most useful. These combinations are best used in draining toxins such as petroleum, radiation, heavy metals and other pollutants because of the drainage effect of the multiple potencies, but they will not bring about permanent changes in biochemistry unless the undesirable state was caused by the body's reaction to the original pollutant. In these cases, draining the toxins allows the body to return to its original state of balanced normality. However, if the original state of the body before the toxin was introduced was unbalanced, removing the toxin will not correct the original problem.

If the body is functioning properly, elimination will be a natural process that will take place automatically. The body has amazing abilities to "detox" on its own without help if allowed to do so. Unless the condition is incurable, single remedies can put these functions back in place.

• What is Health?

We must resist the temptation to view ourselves as unhealthy unless treated. On closer examination, there is no need to believe we are intrinsically sick, and have to be colon cleansed, de-parasited, de-toxed, and over-vitamined to be healthy. While these popular therapies may be called for when there are truly symptoms present that indicate it is necessary, their overuse by symptom free individuals can be harmful. We simply have to allow the body to carry out its natural functions as it is designed to do, gently and easily teaching it if it has lost the knowledge of how to do so.

A single remedy that is well chosen and given in the right potency according to the energy body and level affected, will create an effect that is like a solid board, as a step made of a single plank of wood that will hold up when stepped on and will not fall apart with the first sign of stress.

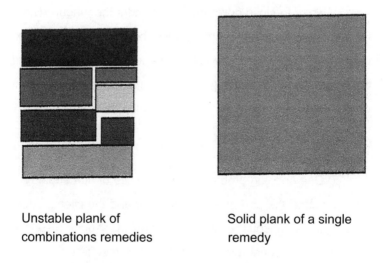

Unstable plank of
combinations remedies

Solid plank of a single
remedy

Figure 9:2 *Single remedies work as a solid plank, stable,
secure and able to bring balance.*

• Single Remedies

Single remedies will do wonderful things if certain principles are followed. First of all, it must be a single remedy taken alone, without any other remedy being mixed with it, or mixed with other single remedies in the mouth while taking it. Other single remedies can be taken close to the same time, but not in the same mouthful.

If a person desires to take more than one single remedy in a short period of time, it is a simple process to do so. First, take the remedy, wait 15 minutes for it to absorb into the portal and the appropriate energy body. Next, eat something or drink a sip of water to close down the portal under the tongue. Then, wait another 15 minute time period before taking the next remedy. In this way, the two single remedies will not mix, and the beneficial effect of using complementary single remedies in quick succession will be achieved and will work well.

• Impatience

One ongoing problem in the practice of homeopathy is impatience on the part of the practitioner and the client. Often, seeking instantaneous results, a client will insist upon a second dose or an additional remedy before allowing sufficient time for the first remedy to fully manifest its actions.

In other cases, a practitioner, perhaps new to the field of homeopathy or desperately wishing to help a client in distress will be tempted to prescribe many remedies simultaneously or in a very short period of time. This is almost always a mistake.

When a remedy is taken, it should not be repeated during its duration of action. Each remedy has its own duration of action. It is the remedy that determines how long it will act--it is not determined by the potency, although 6X potencies are not affected by remedy duration. Even if the symptoms return or increase during the duration of action, the remedy may still be present and acting. It is important to remember that a well-chosen remedy can often produce an aggravation (an increase in symptoms) as it pushes the problem or condition out of the body and energy bodies.

• If Symptoms Return

In a case where there is incomplete clearing of the problem or a short period where the problem was cleared but then returns as before, one should suspect that the remedy was correct, but the potency was wrong. Symptoms return because the potency is incorrect and working on the wrong energy level--not because the remedy has stopped working or has been interrupted by a gross material substance.

Different potencies will work on different energy levels, but it is the remedy that will work over a period of time. For some remedies it is one day, others work for a week or two. Most of the multi-symptom, deep acting constitutional remedies work for 30 to 60, even 90 days. Even if symptoms return, the remedy should not be repeated during this duration, nor should the practitioner hurry to select an additional remedy unless new symptoms indicate the use of a different remedy.

R. Gibson Miller had compiled a chart which gives the duration of action information. This chart is located in the back of the Indian publications (B. Jain Publishers LTD of India) of Boericke's Materia Medica (pages 1079 to 1097), and Kent's Repertory of the Materia Medica (pages 1437 to 1455).

• Lower Potency

No matter what potency is given, do not repeat the same remedy in a lower potency. The energy of the lower potency will fall through the higher potency and cause both to drain out of the body. This can be true for the entire duration of the remedy. If one wishes to repeat a remedy within its duration, go to the next higher potency, never lower.

If, as in the case of calcium absorption, one uses the 30th potency and wishes to switch to the 6X of the same remedy, it is important to remember to use other remedies in between the two potencies of the same substance. If another remedy is used in between the two potencies of the same remedy, the rule for never going to a lower potency in the same remedy does not apply. Lycopodium is often a good remedy choice for this purpose.

In those cases where symptoms go away for a while, but come back unchanged in a short time, the indication is that the potency was too high and went to an energy body and level above the problem, giving temporary amelioration. This can be likened to mowing the lawn to get rid of dandelions. It may remove all of the yellow flowers, but they will simply return because the plant is still present. It was the right remedy, just the wrong potency. It is appropriate to give a complementary remedy before giving the first remedy again in a lower potency. It is not appropriate to repeat the remedy in a lower potency without offsetting its action with a complementary remedy first.

You will find complements of remedies listed in the Miller chart with the duration of action information in the back of Boericke's Materia Medica and Kent's Repertory, but only if it is the book published by B. Jain Publications in India. The books published by Boericke and Tafel in Santa Rose, California do not carry this information.

• Remedy Antidotes

You will also find a list of remedy antidotes in the Miller chart. These refer to potentized antidotes. Gross material chemical-based substances will not antidote a homeopathically potentized remedy--simply because they do not act on the same energy level. If a remedy has stopped working, it has not come in contact with an antidote. It has been given in the wrong potency.

Since the homeopaths of the past have never addressed potency interaction on energy bodies, it seemed reasonable for them to blame outside interference by certain substances as the reason why remedies stopped working. Even today, it is not uncommon to hear one may not use coffee, caffeine, chocolate, camphor, eucalyptus, mint and a variety of other strong smelling substances while using a homeopathic remedy. If it were true that all the prohibitions imposed by these practitioners were actually factors in antidoting remedies, no one would have benefited from homeopathy during its long history. The reality is that chemicals and odors do not antidote potentized remedies. Remedies stop working due to incorrect use of potency.

10

Homeopathy & Allopathy

Homeopathy is a word that describes the use of substances chosen for the symptoms they cause to treat disease that displays the same symptoms as the remedy substance. Allopathy describes conventional medicine in that it is a system of using substances to produce an effect different from those produced by the disease being treated. Homeopathy is an alternative healing system that relies on the concept of energy as the controlling and directing force that regulates the health of the living body. Unlike conventional medicine, which relies on the concept of chemistry as the controlling force, homeopathy does not use material substances and is, therefore, free of harmful effects or unintended side effects.

In homeopathy, substances are reduced to their level of energy by the process known as potentization. These potentized substances are then matched to the individual's unique symptom, placed under the tongue where they are absorbed into an energy portal, thereby, entering the energy bodies of the individual, and relieving those symptoms. These specially prepared substances correct the controlling energy allowing the body to bring itself to normal function. This normalization of the body's energy is reflected in the physical body as changes in physiology as the body returns to a state of health.

• Allopathic (conventional) Medicine

Conventional medicine is based upon a system by which the physician "diagnoses the disease", determines the complex of all symptoms which will define the disease and then determines a course of therapies and chemicals (medications) that will control the disease.

By adding together all of the symptoms found in the people who have been diagnosed with this disease, a symptom profile of the disease is created. This "disease complex", based on a compilation of symptoms obtained from all individuals who have been determined to have this disease, is used as a basis for diagnosis in the future. As each new diagnosis is made, unique symptoms from that particular individual are then added into the disease profile. Because this is an ongoing process, it is unlikely any one individual will display all of the symptoms found in the disease complex. Nor is it unusual to find a symptom in the disease complex which has been discovered in relatively few of the sufferers. A physician will determine the presence of this particular disease in any one individual by looking for any of the symptoms found in the disease complex.

Once this "disease complex" has been established, a physician will continue to use its therapeutic profile for each and every case in which "the disease" has been discovered. All individuals diagnosed with this disease are treated with the same medications regardless of the individuality of their symptoms. In conventional medicine, an individual is often treated for symptoms they do not have and may, therefore, suffer undesirable side effects.

As people who have been diagnosed with this disease and treated with medications develop new symptoms, these are also added into the disease profile and additional medications are found to control these new symptoms. It is an unfortunate fact that many of the "new symptoms" are actual side effects of the previously prescribed medications and that additional "new symptoms" will continue to appear with each additional medication. As this process continues, the disease profile constantly expands and the treatment regime becomes more complex.

• Based on the Energy Fields

Homeopathic medicine, on the other hand, is based solely on the study of a remedy's effect on the energy fields of the individual. In homeopathic medicine, it is the remedy which is placed under constant scrutiny. This study is referred to as a proving. During a proving, healthy individuals take a remedy repeatedly over a short period of time in order to display the energy signature of the remedy. These signatures are identified by the symptoms they produce. The individual conducting the proving records all symptoms that occur. Each and every symptom which a remedy can produce is carefully noted and listed under that remedy's profile. It is as a result of these provings that the remedy's actions on the energetic fields can be determined. As more and more provings are conducted, the full range of the remedy's action can be documented.

• Compare

Homeopathy works by eliminating the symptoms the person is displaying. In homeopathy an individual is never treated for symptoms they do not have regardless of what the disease complex indicates. It is not necessary nor is it advantageous in the practice of homeopathy to attempt to "diagnose the disease" in order to treat the individual. The practitioner need only come to a full and complete understanding of the symptoms displayed by the individual for treatment to be effective.

In conventional medicine, the physician looks at the disease complex and attempts to find the standard treatment for that disease. That standard treatment is designed to eliminate all the symptoms of the disease whether or not they are present in this particular individual. Often the choice of medication is extremely limited as the complexity of symptoms defies a single drug solution. Attempts to use multiple drugs to treat all symptoms have the added problem of drug interaction and unintended side effects.

In addition, because conventional medicine is dedicated to discovering the cause of the disease, it is often difficult or impossible to treat the symptoms before the disease is diagnosed. Many patients spend years looking for the "correct diagnosis" before treatment can begin. Often a diagnosis of a disease for which no standard treatment has been determined will result in the person being told "nothing can be done". In other cases, because the physician is unable to match the symptoms to a known disease complex, the individual is told "you are not really sick, it is all in your head" and no treatment is offered. In these cases, physicians may resort to tranquilizers or mood elevators and label the person a "hypochondriac".

Homeopathic treatment is based upon symptoms displayed by the individual and, therefore, has the choice of many remedies which can work to eliminate those symptoms. The individual is not treated for symptoms they do not display even if those symptoms are listed for the disease. Nor are they denied treatment because there is no diagnosis or because this particular condition has not previously been encountered by the practitioner.

• Choice Vs. Non-option

As an energy medicine, homeopathy represents a choice by the body. Unlike "non-option" treatments such as drugs, chiropractic manipulation, herbs and acupuncture, which the body must interact with, an incorrectly chosen homeopathic remedy is simply ignored by the body's energy fields. Homeopathic remedies cannot be used to force the body to act against its best interests. Homeopathic remedies cannot be used for a "high", nor can they be used to terminate pregnancy or committee suicide.

Doctors and practitioners using conventional drug therapy must deal with the "non-option" aspect of their particular field. No matter how carefully the physician evaluates a case and chooses a course of action, unintended problems can occur. Incorrectly chosen drugs can react with the body in ways that may be fatal. Even the correct drug in excessive doses may be fatal. Chiropractic adjustments "incorrectly done" can result in injury, paralysis or death. Acupuncture, although considered an energy medicine, forces the body to readjust its energy flows as directed by the acupuncturist.

Homeopathic practitioners have the unique advantage of being the field of "option" healing. The body can decide to use the energy of a remedy or simply ignore it. It is this "option" that gives homeopathy its unique safely. Even in extremely large doses, such as an unsupervised child eating the entire contents of a bottle of a homeopathic remedy, there is no adverse effect. This child may get a small reaction to the sugar content of the remedy, but will not suffer from the effects of the remedy itself.

• Chemical Side Effects

Because of the attempt by conventional medicine to treat all possible symptoms of the disease, many medications have chemical components which are intended to treat aspects of the disease that an individual may not have. In addition, many medications are so powerful that they possess the ability to alter the body's chemistry in ways that are not anticipated by the physician. These unintended alterations in the body's chemistry and functions are commonly referred to as side effects. Many symptoms originally thought of as part of the disease complex may actually be side effects of the medication used to treat the original condition.

Homeopathic remedies are energetic in nature and, therefore, cannot have side effects. These remedies will not create symptoms or conditions in a person which are not already present, nor can they be used to create an action or condition beyond the normal range of the individual. Homeopathic medicines can only eliminate symptoms which are already present or establish balance in nutrient absorption and distribution. Because of this action, treating an individual with homeopathic medicines cannot produce the additional problems often associated with conventional medicines.

• Homeopathy is <u>Not</u> for Every Case

Homeopathy is a system which assists the body in healing. It is not a "fast" medicine and cannot be used in cases where "time is of the essence" such as automobile accidents, broken bones or accidental poisonings. Homeopathy will not replace "non-option" medicine in cases where it is the most appropriate choice. <u>Attempting to use homeopathy in all situations is both short-sighted and reckless and does a disservice to both the client and the practitioner</u>. The value of homeopathy, when used correctly, is without question. <u>When used incorrectly, homeopathy is at best worthless, and in the worse case, may delay appropriate treatment until the individual suffers permanent and irreversible harm, up to and including death.</u>

It is extremely important to remember that homeopathy is considered a complementary medicine and is effective when used in conjunction with other forms of treatment. <u>Homeopathy does not stand in opposition to conventional medicine and can be used to assist the body in recovering from surgery, dental</u>

procedures and other forms of treatments. Many of the side effects caused by the appropriate use of necessary medications can be treated by using homeopathic remedies without the fear that these remedies will interact with the medications.

Homeopathy differs from herbal medicine in safely when used with conventional medicine. Herbal remedies, often touted as the safe and effective choice, can and will interact with the body and other forms of "non-option" medicines such as drugs. These reactions are often unknown and unpredictable and, therefore, beyond the ability of the practitioner to prevent.

Homeopathy can be used to enhance a person's optimal health by bringing the body into complete balance. It is not a system of "super nutrition", nor is it a method by which the body can be forced to exceed its natural limits. Homeopathy does not expand an individual's optimum range, but rather allows the individual to reach their optimum level of health. Understanding and accepting the natural limits of the body is vitally important to preserving the health and well being of the individual. Failure to understand and accept that the body has natural predetermined limits can result in a person taking action which damages or destroys the individual's health.

Ultimately, what you don't know about your body may lead to action that could cause permanent harm.

11

Compensation Illnesses

In modern society, there is a tendency to want our bodies and minds to function beyond normal human capabilities. The idea of becoming "Superman" invulnerable to pain, disease, stress or any of the other normal life occurrences has been hailed as the only acceptable form of human existence. This unreachable and unrealistic model is held forth as a goal for which one must continually strive or else be viewed as somehow "less".

In this quest, many people are looking to herbs and other substances they have been told will help them achieve this "ideal" goal. Unfortunately, many people also believe that as long as the substance they are using is "natural" everything will be okay--that a "natural substance" can be used without any danger or thought as to its true effect on the body. Herbs, vitamins, minerals, and hormones are all consumed at levels far exceeding the body's ability to utilize or process these substances. Because they are deemed natural, many people believe that no harmful effects can come from their over utilization. In actual fact, this belief can lead an individual to actions that eventually result in diminished health or actual illness. In worse case scenarios, the over utilization of a "natural substance" can lead to death.

• Herbs as Medicine

An often overlooked aspect in medicine is that herbs represented the original pharmacopoeia with which the doctor treated his patients. The rise of industrial chemistry allowed the drug companies to duplicate these chemicals on a wide scale basis without resorting to harvesting and extracting the chemical from the original plant. This division into chemically produced substances and "natural herbs" has led people to believe that herbs are somehow "safe supplements" and prescription, or over-the-counter medications are "drugs".

In reality, the major difference between herbs and drugs lies in the concentration levels of the chemical and the consistency of that chemical. Naturally grown herbs can and will vary in their chemical composition as a result of their growing conditions, techniques used for harvesting and processing as well as the length of time in storage. The reality is that herbs work like chemicals in the body and force changes in the body's chemistry.

In addition, herbal substances are often chosen for one aspect rather than considering the full range of their action. Herbs such as Ma Huang (Ephedra), Ginkgo Biloba and Ginseng are stimulants which force the body to work harder than normal. Because people make the assumption that these "natural" stimulants are free of the side effects found in "chemical" stimulants, they will often choose to use them even when they would never consider taking any form of "speed". Many people who have been told by their doctors that they must avoid caffeine, diet pills, and other forms of chemical stimulants, will select these herbs as a replacement because they provide the body with "natural energy". In actual fact, these "natural" stimulants also wear out the adrenal glands just as "chemical" stimulants do, which results in continuous fatigue in the long run.

• Displacement

A second aspect of chemical medications that is often overlooked is referred to as "displacement". Displacement occurs when the body begins to substitute the chemicals being consumed for those it would have made on its own. Displacement is a result of the conservation of energy by the body. Basically, from the body's viewpoint, why expend the energy creating a chemical which is clearly abundant and available from the environment?

Stimulants such as amphetamines and ephedrine all displace the natural energy chemicals of the body. When these chemicals are stopped, the person is literally unable to get out of bed. A common example is the addiction to pain relievers, prescription or otherwise. When a person habitually uses pain killers such as aspirin or opiates the body begins to use these drugs to suppress pain and stops making the natural endorphins which would otherwise have helped suppress the pain. This displacement is a contributing factor to the inability of a person to "break their addiction". When a person addicted to a pain killer stops taking the medication, their body is without the chemical and is no longer capable of producing it on its own. As a result, the person is in more pain than a person who did not habitually use pain killers.

Recovery from this type of addiction is very difficult as the body does not immediately resume the production of the missing chemicals. Indeed, it may take several years for the body to begin to produce these chemicals on its own. Relapse into addiction often occurs as the person continues to need the drugs they are no longer taking and cannot produce on their own.

• The Perfect Man

The idea that everyone is less than perfect can be traced in the medical literature as far back as Plato. In Plato's time, the concept of the ideal, that original state of perfection that each person was innately aware of was heralded as the model for all aspects of life that one should strive to obtain. Each being was considered to be an imperfect copy of the ideal state of perfection who longed to return to that state. It was therefore believed everyone could reach that ideal state if only they received the needed corrections and enhancements.

This idea has been passed through the generations and continues to operate in today's society. Advertising agencies, self-development programs and personal enhancement trainers all rely on this concept. When compared to the "original intended state of perfection" or today's models, everyone falls short. Everyone has some form of illness and no one is truly healthy. Even if a person believes himself to be okay, he is often viewed as living in a state of denial and told that he is "just fooling himself". If he continues to insist that there is nothing wrong, he is then told there are many ways to exceed his personal limits, expand his horizons and go beyond those limits to reach levels he never believed were possible.

Many ways to reach these goals are described and prescribed by the advocates of these systems. Herbs can be used to enhance performance and provide the body with energy reserves allowing intense physical training. A therapist can always find flaws in personality which are causes of self-sabotage and allow us to fall short of our goals. A doctor can always find some condition for which medication will be helpful along with some future disease or problem which can be prevented only by adhering to a specific diet, taking certain supplements or engaging in specific forms of physical activity. While some modifications in the typical "modern" lifestyle may be beneficial to some people, much of what is now being hyped as beneficial promises results beyond what is reasonable for any person to believe.

An example of this belief is easily seen when looking at how we now view mental functions. In order to compete in today's modern society, people are required to understand and retain vast amounts of ever changing information. As this information overload continues, people begin to question why it is impossible for them to have full command of all the "facts at hand". Instead of questioning whether all the information is truly necessary or processing it into forms or concepts that allow the information to be used, people are told that their memory is not good enough, that they may be suffering various forms of failure, or that their memory could be better. The herb Ginkgo Biloba has been touted as a "cure" for this all too often non-existent problem.

In their effort to remain a functional part of today's competitive society, people are flocking to health food stores to stock up on Ginkgo. Many have no identifiable problems, but believe they must take Ginkgo regardless of the present state of their memory in order to maintain their "edge". Although Ginkgo may be appropriate for use in a person whose memory is failing as a result of some forms of circulation impairment, there is no evidence it will enhance a person's memory beyond their normal limitations.

Ginkgo is an herb that has been reported to increase the blood flow to the cranial area, thereby, bringing more oxygen and nutrients to the brain cells. It is hoped that this added blood flow will help to improve a person's memory. The problem with the over use, or inappropriate use, of this substance lies within the very action that is touted as beneficial. Ginkgo works by pushing more blood into the blood vessels than would normally be present. This can raise blood pressure, trigger migraine headaches, or lead to stroke in weakened blood vessels.

An underlying problem, often not mentioned or even considered, is that the inappropriate use of Ginkgo can trigger the body to compensate and fight back against this new change in status. The body has mechanisms to counteract what it perceives as problems, i.e., sudden changes in what has been the "normal" functioning of the body. When a person quits using Ginkgo, these compensation mechanisms continue to function because they are now the normal state of the body. Without the continual stimulation of the Ginkgo, the circulation to the brain can slow down to levels below its pre-Ginkgo norm, thereby, creating an entirely new set of problems which now need to be "corrected".

• Human Limits

Our bodies are designed to function in the normal range and must be allowed to rest when tired. Artificial attempts to surpass those limits, whether by use of "natural substances" or "chemical substances", are damaging to our overall health. We cannot continually go beyond our innate limits and not expect to pay for those excesses in the long run.

It is important to change the mindset of people in today's society. Time and time again it has been proven that trying to make something function beyond its normal limitations is asking for trouble. People accept these limitations in all aspects of their life, except where their body is concerned. Cars, lawn mowers, blenders and mechanical devices are maintained and used within their limits. People understand and accept that overusing these devices will result in their breakdown and failure. Yet, where their bodies, which must last a lifetime, are concerned, people continue to believe that they can ignore the limits with impunity.

People must come to understand and embrace the normal functioning of the body. Instead of constantly trying to over enhance what nature has designed the human body to do, people must allow it to function as it was designed. Normal balance and optimum health should be the goal.

- ## Memory

A person who is believed to be suffering a memory problem, may instead be experiencing a biochemical imbalance, a problem with energy flow, or an emotional upset, all of which can create such a distraction that the person is unable to think clearly. Ginkgo Biloba will only stimulate the blood flow and cannot correct any of these additional problems. A person using Ginkgo and finding no relief may become even more desperate as the promised cure fails to occur. Often they will increase the amount of the herb, hoping somehow that an additional amount will solve the problem. The additional stress, both physical from the chemical action of the herb, and mental from the failure of the cure, simply increases the "memory problem".

The homeopathic approach to treating this same "memory problem" would involve asking the person to describe their symptoms. By so doing, underlying stresses, imbalances and other causative factors would be detected. Additionally, other symptoms in the body, such as digestive disorders, sleep problems or grief issues, not treated by Ginkgo because they were not deemed part of the memory problem, would also be corrected. A homeopathically prepared substance reduced to energy (this concept is more fully elaborated on in the following text) and properly matched to the symptoms can gently correct the problem--permanently--rather than covering it up with a gross substance that can create an additional problem.

For example, a person showing signs of what is commonly known as Alzheimer's may have some damage in the brain due to falls and accidents. Homeopathic remedies can help heal the damage. There may be some accumulation of heavy metals such as zinc, aluminum and lead clouding mental function, all of which can be drained homeopathy. Finally, mental functions can be enhanced with simple, safe homeopathic doses, bringing the person back from a devastating problem. This is a course of action that takes time and effort on the part of the client and the practitioner, but the results of very gratifying.

The knowledge of homeopathy is coming back into consciousness in today's society as the limitations of conventional medicine become more apparent. Although there exists significant misunderstanding and many incorrect assumptions, careful study will clarify the system and its proper use. There is a simple method by which the true nature of homeopathy and how the system is used to enhance the health of the individual that can easily be learned enabling homeopathy to be used by individuals from every walk of life. Read on--this system appears later in the book.

12

Failure to Nourish Illnesses

The human body is made up of billions of tiny biological units, each alive as a separate entity that eats, metabolizes, excretes, reproduces and dies. Each of these individual cells has requirements of nutrition to keep them healthy and functioning properly. If the receptor sites on the cell membrane are reduced in number or unable to recognize certain nutrients as good food and something useful, the cell will not take in enough of the food for its need. If a large number of cells in the body fail to recognize a nutrient as necessary, the entire body will feel the stress of deficiency. The fluid between the cells may be awash with these nutrients, but the cells have to take it in and use it on a large scale for the body to be relieved of the stress of deficiency. The most common minerals the body will have problems absorbing are calcium, magnesium, silica, sulfur and salt.

The easiest way for cells to recognize a nutrient is for the particular nutrient molecule to be partially converted to an energetic form by the potentizing process of converting material into homeopathic form. Homeopathic processes begin the conversion of the material substance into its energetic form. Often the substances in the body cannot be converted into an energetic form because the body lacks sufficient vital energy to begin the conversion of that particular substance.

In some cases, the body has sufficient vital force to convert a small amount of the substance, but lacks sufficient force to convert an adequate amount. This can be compared to trying to start a fire with only charcoal. At some point a match or other ignition source must be used to begin the original fire.

In other cases, there is a small fire but it is insufficient to light the larger pieces of material and is, therefore, extinguished when the larger pieces are added. Homeopathically prepared materials function much as a lighter and lighter fluid in starting these necessary conversion processes.

• Calcium

Calcium is a nutrient that is so important in the human body that it controls the body's response to infection. When a person is calcium deficient, infection is a life-long problem and can be life-threatening without antibiotics.

Calcium also is used by the body to heal injury--not just broken bones, but brain trauma and deep tissue wounds as well. More obviously, calcium holds up the body by strengthening the skeletal structures. We have seen the results of skeletal calcium loss in sufferers of rickets and osteoporosis.

Many people believe that taking the gross material form is all that is needed to prevent the problems associated with deficiencies. Often people will say, "I take calcium, a 1000 mg a day, I can't be calcium deficient". This statement simply reflects the confusion between what is taken into the body and what can be used by the body. Gross form calcium, no matter how much is present in the body, may not be used properly until it is converted into its energetic form.

The actual situation in most cases is that calcium in its gross whole molecular form is so large the cells of the body perceive it as a foreign object. This inability of the cells to recognize calcium as a nutrient occurs for many people in the U.S. due to the fact that we are the descendants of immigrants to this country. Those of us whose ancestors emigrated from the British Isles countries, the Northern European areas of Belgium and The Netherlands, the fish eating coastal cultures of Europe, Mexico, and Polynesia are descendants from biological bodies that were accustomed to large amounts of iodine in the food source. The difference in the iodine levels in the food interrupts the production of thyroid hormones which interrupts the hormones of the parathyroid gland, which in turn interrupts the conversion of calcium to an energy form and absorption into cells. Once this pathway has been interrupted, it does not bounce back to normal easily and usually requires help.

The residents of the British Isles countries, particularly Ireland, seem to be prone to this problem due to the fact that their ancestors used sea kelp to fertilize the agricultural fields. The switch to modern fertilizers or the import of food from other countries will produce the same iodine deficiency in modern day residents of these areas as it does for residents in the U.S.

The cells will not allow this calcium molecule to pass through the receptor sites on the outer cell membrane or the body lacks sufficient vital force to convert the calcium molecule into energy. In most cases, the calcium an individual takes in supplements just sits in the intercellular fluids and starts to deposit in nodules and around joints, which causes a new set of problems. Recent research indicates the overuse of calcium supplements in women causes fibroid tumors and in men contributes to the arthritic overgrowth of calcium in the joints.

If people have calcium deposits where they shouldn't have them, a doctor is very likely to take them off all forms of calcium, which doesn't solve the calcium deficiency problem or correct the problem with calcium deposits. In most cases, the deficiency caused by iodine interruption does not register as a calcium deficiency by any test doctors now have available to them. Currently, there is no way to test the calcium level inside cells of tissue. This is the reason why this calcium deficiency problem goes undetected by conventional medicine.

Only the homeopathically prepared dose of calcium, Calcarea Carb. or Calcarea Phos., can open the door of the receptor sites of the individual cells and allow calcium to get in- -as well as teach the body how to get rid of the excess, bringing balance. Only a homeopathically prepared dose of calcium can begin the conversion of gross form calcium to energetic calcium necessary to make solid the energy bodies.

Over the years, I have often seen children with frequent ear infections, tonsillitis or some other frequently occurring infection as a result of calcium deficiency. When presented with these symptoms the first thing I think of is homeopathic calcium. Upon beginning a regime of Calcium based remedies, Calcarea Carb. followed by a couple of months on Calcarea Phos., these children are able to completely get rid of these recurring infections.

A head trauma patient who has seizures due to damaged brain tissue stops having seizures and begins to heal with homeopathic calcium.

Adult patients who have a life long history of infections- -tonsil, ear, sinus or lung--and as an adult have digestion and stomach problems--and often with sleep problems--can change many things with homeopathic calcium. People suffering from low levels of constant pain--who often say "I don't really hurt but I just don't feel good" often find relief after taking homeopathic calcium.

Children and adults who are a bit sluggish, have a tendency to be overweight and have poor muscle tone will have no control over what they eat because their calcium starved tissues cry out to be fed. It is as if the billions of individual cells crying out in unison create a fear of starvation. Without proper nutrient absorption, cells surrounded by calories will still feel deprived.

• Sodium Chloride

Another problem nutrient is salt, sodium chloride. Do you know someone who craves salty foods--potato chips, snack foods, french fries etc.--and can't seem to get enough? It seems strange so many people crave something that is so harmful when used to excess. Yet when homeopathic principles are understood, the explanation becomes surprisingly clear. The individual cells are not getting enough of the sodium chloride they need. There is a block to cell absorption. The cells cry out for sodium because they can't get it. All the salt the person is eating sits in the intercellular fluid, piling up and causing problems such as dehydration in the tissues, a lessening of spinal fluid, and high pressure in the blood vessels due to the attraction of fluid from tissue into the high sodium concentration flowing in the vessels.

The homeopathic preparation of salt, Natrum Muriaticum--is sodium chloride potentized and converted to an energy form which can enter the cells and relieve the deficiency.

I treated a four-year-old boy once who was whinny, pale, thin and anemic (diagnosed anemic by his doctor), and unable to speak clearly. He used only two words at a time, and even those words were not easily understood. I gave him a three-day-course of Nat.Mur in the 30th potency. Four weeks later, I saw a lively, happy, playful boy, who was not thin, not pale, not sickly-- and according to his regular doctor, no longer anemic. He was speaking better and using words more clearly. I couldn't believe he was the same child.

Anemia is a problem for the sodium deficient person because the bones will be sodium deficient and lacking proper moisture. Bones that are dry and brittle may not produce bone marrow that can form red blood cells correctly. These red blood cells may not be able to carry enough iron and hemoglobin required by the body, leading to anemia. The problem is not the lack of iron often, but rather the ability of the blood cells to carry proper amounts.

I saw a six-month-old baby recently with a broken leg. The mother explained that the baby had fallen from the bed and his leg had snapped. I was astounded. A baby of only six months of age should not have bones brittle enough to break so easily.

It seemed obvious to me this baby had a sodium absorption problem which would translate to more difficult problems as the baby grew.

It was Natrum Mur. in a single dose of 200C, the appropriate potency for the mental level for his age, that eliminated the symptoms of Autism for my son when he was two years old. Autism, in its classical manifestation, is a sodium chloride deficiency in the cells of the brain that prevents the development of certain skills and the processing of information in children who are deficient. Always, these children will crave salty food.

• The Sodium Constitution

In some people, the bones may be too dry and brittle to absorb calcium correctly due to a lack of sodium chloride absorption into the bone structures of the body. For these people, it is necessary to complete a regime of homeopathic sodium chloride remedies to make sure the bones are moist enough to take in new calcium. Natrum Muriaticum is the main remedy for this purpose.

A person with a need to balance sodium, a Natrum Mur. constitution, will be a person who craves salty foods and adds a lot of salt to their food, or would have a desire to add salt even though they have been told not to.

This person would be thirsty, because the body is trying to put moisture in the places where it is needed, but in reality, the moisture does not go where it should and can accumulate where it shouldn't. This excess moisture can be in the form of edema, or what used to be called dropsy. This person may even have high blood pressure due to the amount of sodium and fluid in the blood, yet the bones and brain tissue will go without. The bones become dry and brittle. Very often this person is anemic, since lack of moisture in the long bones where the marrow is producing red blood cells makes it impossible for the marrow to produce blood cells correctly.

The mind of the Natrum Mur. constitution has problems processing information and keeping memory intact due to the lack of sodium. It is sodium chloride as a chemical in brain tissue that helps the brain process information and put that information into files, the same way a computer works, to make it available for memory. Without proper amounts of that chemical, the system malfunctions.

This person may have a life-long problem with learning disabilities. This is the student with a noticeable problem in learning to read where the person hated school and avoided going to college. Sometimes it is more subtle. The person who does not read for pleasure because it is not easy or pleasurable and yet managed to graduate from college with a professional degree may have a sodium absorption problem as well. This is probably the student who had to spend a lot of time in the books compared to other students who got their reading done more quickly and remembered the information easily.

Children with a salt craving are also in this situation. These children will have a problem with learning to read, assimilating and processing what they read and will probably hate school. Natrum Mur. remedies will change the entire situation for these kids, hopefully before they reach an age where it is no longer possibly to change the destiny of their career.

Many people are born with a sodium absorption problem, but it can also be acquired through extreme grief. Grief is a situation that interferes with sodium absorption. Many people who have experienced a grief event, or a highly emotional situation, will suddenly become salt cravers. From that point on, the brain will not be able to process information correctly and the person loses interest in life or studies. They may develop headaches from eye strain, begin to have trouble relating to people, and eventually will develop anemia or high blood pressure. The longer this situation goes on the more severe it becomes.

The accumulation of grief over a lifetime intensifies all of these problems, which manifests as the common symptoms and weakness of old age and senility, which is considered normal. It doesn't have to be that way.

When given the sodium remedies, people stop craving salt, the mind processes the grief information and people go on with their lives without physical changes, as long as it has not been long enough for damage to have caused permanent tissue change.

I just finished reading an article in the newspaper dated November 4, 2004, suggesting that inflammatory gut disease may be the cause of autism in some children. What is not understood is that the inflammatory gut disease problem and autism are both caused by the same condition, a lack of absorption of sodium chloride into the cells of body tissue. Both conditions can be present in the individual in need of Natrum Mur. as a homeopathic remedy. It is important to understand that the inflammation of the intestines is not a cause of a secondary condition, but rather a symptom of the same situation that allows both conditions to occur.

• Other Nutrients

An individual suffering from a deficiency of sulfur as a nutrient may experience dry mucus membranes and recurring sinus infections. These sinus infections are due to the lack of proper viscosity of body fluids and an inability of the mucus membranes to produce enough mucus to allow the sinuses to clear properly. It is the viscosity of body fluids that is regulated by the nutrient sulfur. This is often the situation that leads to uncomfortable symptoms during the time of menopause. Interestingly, menopause is often a time when a woman may experience more sinus infections than at other times in her life.

The symptoms of a deficiency of magnesium may include muscle cramping, arthritic type symptoms, migraine headaches that occur with cycles of the menstrual period and a lowered resistance which may inhibit the body's ability to ward off cancer cell growth.

A person suffering from silica deficiency may have hair, nail or skin problems which may manifest as fungus and bacterial infection due to lack of resistance. This person may also feel as if they cannot stand up against life and experience an inability to make decisions.

We as human beings cannot expect to live beyond what is a normal lifetime for our organic bodies, but perhaps we can be healthy, in proper functioning condition and mentally coherent until our time is up. The founder of homeopathy, Samuel Hahnemann, was all of that when he died of an acute lung infection in his 90's in the late nineteenth century--at a time when life expectancy was around 50 years of age. It is important to recognize the fact that human bodies are energetically motivated and animated. Ignoring this fact allows deficiencies to continue.

13

Degenerative Illnesses

Degenerative illnesses are those acquired in life from physical activity that results in overuse or continuous use of a body part. Conditions such as arthritis, carpal tunnel, jogger's knee and tennis elbow are a few examples. Degenerative illnesses manifest in an area that is already weakened or has an underlying condition which allows the problem to occur.

Motion that is repeated continuously over a period of time creates an overuse in one set of muscles and a corresponding under use in the complementary muscle set. At the same time, this continual use of a small isolated section of the body can deplete that segment of one or more of the vital nutrients necessary for balanced function.

In this small and localized area, the deficiency may create a syndrome which the body does not have time to correct. This can occur for several reasons. In many cases, the continual use of a nutrient normally present in the body in minute quantities depletes the overall reserve which cannot be replenished by the body. It is equally important to note that depleting these vital nutrients can result in pain and dysfunction not necessarily isolated to the area suffering the over use.

• Blood Flow Problems

In other cases, the blood flow into an area that is in continual use is inadequate to meet the body's demands, resulting in deficit conditions which the body could correct given sufficient time. Unfortunately, the time needed to rebalance these deficit conditions may exceed what the person's "work" schedule allows creating a situation in which deficit is continually expanding. It is important to note that these deficit conditions may include properties not normally considered by allopathic medicine. Examples of this include cooling, heating, lubrication, pressure and other aspects of mechanical function.

In addition, the body's attempts to isolate the area or limit the movements by that muscle group in order to allow sufficient time for healing can create pain, stiffness, weakness or other feelings of discomfort. As a result, the person may shift the functions normally performed by that area to the opposite side resulting in overuse and damage to the previously good corresponding area. For example, an injury to one knee may result in the person limping and standing with their weight on the opposite leg, damaging that leg as well. As a result of the misalignment of the body, the person may also develop back pain and headaches. As the problem is allowed to continue, more and more of the body begins to suffer, both from the depletion of vital nutrients and the continual shifting of body functions to undamaged or lesser damaged areas.

• Protection

Giving an appropriate homeopathic remedy allows the body to replace or redistribute the vital nutrients much more quickly. By having the appropriate nutrients available in their energetic form, the body is able to create solid energy fields which protect the area from further damage. In addition, by intercepting the illness or damage in its earliest form these compensation efforts, i.e., the shifting of use to the corresponding opposite areas, and the resulting progression of damage and pain throughout the body, can be prevented.

• Carpal Tunnel Syndrome

Carpal Tunnel Syndrome results from activities in which only the wrist and finger control muscles move. The carpal area is a fixed diameter passage through which the tendons and nerves going to the fingers must pass. With continual overuse, these muscles and tendons get inflamed and expand beyond normal levels creating constriction and jamming of the tendons. As a person continues to use their hands, the tendons and carpal area become torn and damaged resulting in more and more pain and less and less function. The resulting constriction and jamming also deprives the muscles and tendons of vital nutrients because although blood flows easily into relaxed muscles, it cannot flow as easily into those in use or damaged.

Homeopathic treatment for the symptoms described by the individual and matched to the proper remedy would target the area of the problem, bring about a balance of nutrients and a strengthening of the energy fields, thereby, allowing the body to correct the problem. However, it is important to note that if the damage has gone beyond the body's ability to correct the problem on its own, the homeopathic remedy will not succeed.

There is some medical evidence to suggest that lowered thyroid function and resulting calcium deficiency plays a part in carpel tunnel problems.

• Repetitive Movement Injury

A repetitive movement injury is caused over time. Activities such as lifting items over and over, repeatedly bending the elbow, overusing the shoulder, and straining the back are a few examples. Lack of proper nutrients also creates a condition which slowly penetrates the energy bodies, creating a weakened area in the physical body and a corresponding gap in the lower energy levels. It is extremely important to note that both of these conditions are extrusive and push from the inside out. These conditions require a lower potency in the remedy, given over a longer period of time to reverse the condition because of the time it took for the problem to develop.

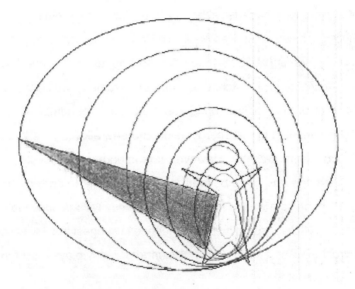

Figure 13:1 Overuse injury starts inside the body and
            penetrates outward.

Degenerative conditions caused by chronic overuse and improper nutrient levels can result in conditions in the body which allow traumatic events to occur. For example, long standing calcium deficiencies may result in chronic infections which weaken the body's immune system making the person more susceptible to influenza and communicable diseases. Additionally, chronic calcium shortages can also create bones which lack sufficient strength to deal with day to day life and are, therefore, easily broken, even in the most minor of falls. It can happen that a chronic degenerative problem which began on the physical level will penetrate out through the energy bodies allowing a traumatic injury to occur.

• Sudden Traumatic Injury

Degenerative illnesses or conditions are different from injuries which occur as a result of a traumatic event. Trauma is intrusive and comes from the outside of the body and normally occurs as a result of an extremely fast or instantaneous event. These injuries are acute in nature and rarely begin as a nutrient failure, although improper nutrition may contribute to the severity of the injury. In virtually every case of traumatic injury, the person can pinpoint the exact moment and method by which the injury occurred. Falling from roller blades is not an overuse injury.

A traumatic condition starts from outside and penetrates in. Given sufficient time, any traumatic event will become intrinsic and appear to be a chronic condition. It is important that traumatic events be treated as quickly as possible using a high potency to stop the event from moving into the lower energy bodies and becoming a chronic physical problem.

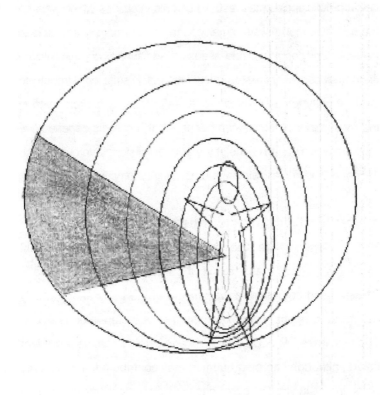

Figure 13:2 Trauma starts from the outer bodies and
penetrates inward over time.

In cases of long standing traumatic injuries, even though
the injury started as a single traumatic event, compensation
efforts by the body will have spread the initial injury over a much
larger area and created chronic degenerative problems in those

areas. For example, a severely sprained ankle can result in a tear in the Achilles tendon. This tear, if allowed to remain untreated, can result in the person limping to avoid the pain in the ankle. Unfortunately, over time, this limp will create excess wear on the hip and knee joint of the opposite leg and can even result in disc rupture in the lower back. The initial injury was traumatic, instantaneous and intrusive, but if left untreated, it will create a degenerative condition which is slow, chronic and extrusive.

Since most degenerative problems affect the skeletal and connective tissue structures of the body, it is appropriate to use the low potencies (6X) of the Schussler Cell Salt Remedies to help with these problems.

14

Inappropriate Learning Diseases

Inappropriate learning diseases are almost always a result of the overuse of substances. In the '70's, research suggested that individuals might ward of the cold and flu virus by taking massive doses of vitamin C. Even symptom free people rushed to the drug stores to stock up, and began using lots of vitamin C, even on a daily basis, just to make sure. A few years later it was decided that C does not stay in the body more than 24 hours, so everyone must take vitamin C, a least 1000mg. everyday just to maintain normal health. What happened before the 1970's that caused people who were healthy and getting along just fine without vitamin C supplements to suddenly need the 1000mg daily--just to survive?

• Vitamin C

By taking large doses of vitamin C, the person creates an overload condition which causes the body to perceive this substance as toxic, since it is present in levels far above what the body can use. The body responds to this condition by systematically and continuously eliminating the vitamin C. The body has no reason to attempt to conserve the vitamin C because it has been taught that massive continual doses will always be forthcoming. When the person stops taking the massive amounts of vitamin C, the body is unable to believe that it is now safe to store the vitamin C. In effect, the body can not immediately unlearn this new lesson, and continues to eliminate the vitamin C no matter how little is now coming in. Previously healthy people now find that when they stop taking their supplements, they become ill and suffer problems which are attributed to vitamin C deficiencies thus convincing them they were correct and the massive doses are necessary. It is easy to understand why people who where tested to see how long vitamin C was in the body, were found free of excess after 24 hours--since the body eliminates excess materials as rapidly as possible to prevent toxic levels. It should be noted that the testing was not conducted to establish if the person had vitamin C deficiencies within 24 hours, only to determine if the body had eliminated the supplemental amounts given for the test. Overuse of substances teaches the body to get rid of it, and the lesson is permanent--unless changed on an energy level.

The English sailors who were found to have scurvy used only a half a lime a day to ward off the problem. It should be noted that these sailors were at sea for years at a time with no other source of vitamin C and, therefore, should not be used as an example of normal nutrition. It is unlikely in today's world that anyone eating a reasonably balanced diet could suffer such severe problems as those found in English sailors of the 1800's. Even in these extreme conditions it was noted that the amount of vitamin C necessary to prevent scurvy was limited to the amount present in one half of a lime. How many milligrams of C is in half a lime; the answer is probably un-measurable by today's mega standards. It's the mega doses that are the problem. People are taking 1500 mg a day when maybe only 50 to 500 mg is the correct amount needed.

It is important to understand that a study based on a single element of the population living in conditions not identical to the average lifestyle cannot be used to establish that a supplement is necessary for everyone. A substance which is beneficial to a limited number of people should not be viewed as an absolute necessity for all people. Nor should a substance deemed harmful for a limited population be view has harmful to all people.

It can be likened to a city that experiences a flood one year and decides to build massive flood control channels so the problem will not happen again. Each time it rains the flood channels work very efficiently to get rid of the excess water. But in a year when rain is normal, the flood channels still work at top efficiency, creating drought.

On another issue, those of us who have been calcium deficient most of our lives may also be in need of a regular dose of vitamin C in order to bring tone and balance to tissue compromised by the inability to absorb calcium in the past. This is a situation which benefits from doses of 100 to 500 mg a day of vitamin C for a period of time in order to help the body restore tone and strength to connective tissue and blood vessels. This amount of vitamin C use will also help curb appetite since the tissues deficient in calcium from the past have probably been unable to absorb vitamin C as well, contributing to the cravings that lead to overeating. However, this condition does not require massive doses of C and one must be cautious not to fall for the wrong advice on the issue.

One condition that may be helped by massive doses of vitamin C on a very limited basis is a condition where environmental toxins are causing a health problem, such as is suspected in MS (Multiple Sclerosis). Doses of 2000 mg for only two or three days has been known to help de-tox suspect toxins from the body. This is the result of the body's need to flush the excess vitamin C to prevent toxicity which acts to flush other toxins suspected to cause other illnesses.

Please note this is an extremely specialized and limited use of high potency dosing of vitamin C. Continuing to take large amounts of vitamin C over a long period of time can damage the lining of blood vessels due to the scouring action of large doses. In turn, higher levels of cholesteral may be produced by the liver to shore up tears in blood vessels, creating new problems.

• Avoiding salt

Another example of inappropriate learning can be found in people who avoid salt. This practice teaches the body to hold onto all salt and the person soon finds they cannot use any salt at all without symptoms. The American diet is high in salt compared to other countries, but eliminating salt completely is not the answer. Sodium chloride is an absolutely necessary nutrient to the body. The body cannot tolerate a salt deficiency and must compensate if salt is being deprived.

• Avoiding Oil

People who eliminate oil from their diet for the sake of dieting to lose weight will teach the body to make cholesterol. In addition, they may begin suffering from diseases caused by the lack of essential fatty acids such as joint pain for lack of lubrication and gall bladder disease. After deficiency is established, the first time the person eats oil, the body overreacts and hordes all the oil, raising the level of fatty acids and cholesterol in the blood, thereby, creating a condition in which the person must constantly monitor their diet to eliminate oils and dietary cholesterol to prevent the elevated cholesterol levels from occurring.

• Overdosing with Vitamins

It is a trend these days to take massive doses of vitamins, antioxidants, vitamin E, lots of the B's--all mixed in with multi-minerals. This practice teaches the body to be very efficient at elimination, and soon, a person must take these things just to stay normal. This is true for Melatonin and DHEA which are naturally occurring hormones. By taking them as supplements, the body stops natural production and eliminates the excess. The process of diminished production and increased elimination continues, even after one stops taking the supplements.

• Be Cautious

Avoid falling into the media hype and advertising that promotes the practice of over-taking vitamins. I once had a question from a person who wondered why she got a headache every time she took a vitamin supplement. She wanted to know what to do about the headache so she could take the vitamins she was convinced were absolutely necessary for "good health". It never occurred to her that her body didn't need or want the vitamins and was using the headache to tell her that taking vitamins was inappropriate. Instead, she insisted on finding a way to stop her body from telling her that following what everyone else said was "necessary" may not be the right thing for her to do.

Become aware of what is really happening and avoid popular trends, particularly when they are new and wonderful. Nothing is that wonderful and there is no fountain of youth. When the newness wears off, problems start to appear.

Homeopathic remedies do not teach inappropriate learning since the substances are diluted and not material enough to be perceived as toxic and eliminated by the body. Massive doses of gross calcium causes problems such as deposits in joints and fibroid uterine tumors, but the homeopathically prepared dose of Calcarea teaches the body to use calcium correctly.

Iron supplements cause problems when the body tries to get rid of the excess. Many people have cramps, constipation, or blood in the stool from taking iron. There is a disease that is due to a toxic overload of iron that can be very dangerous. Homeopathic iron, Ferrum Met. or Ferrum Phos. can teach the body to use iron correctly, and cannot cause overload or symptoms since it is an energy dose. The proper use of homeopathic iron-derived remedies can reduce the occurrence of chronic inflammation in the body, particularly in blood vessels. Chronic inflammation has been suggested to be the cause of stroke and heart attack. Ferrum Phos. in the 6X potency taken over a period of one month is very helpful in reducing chronic inflammation.

• Correcting the Problem

Homeopathically prepared doses of substances that have created inappropriately learned responses can correct the problem by promoting absorption and stopping the elimination. Another way is to simply stop taking the substance. When symptoms of deprivation arise, a remedy matched to the symptoms will help the body pinpoint the problem and correct it.

• Compensation Disease

A compensation disease is one that develops with treatment for a symptom that resulted in unexpected symptoms. For example, my friend with the head trauma took antacids to control seizures. The extra calcium in the stomach produced more acid, since the stomach cannot remain in a neutral state. The creation of more acid meant she had to continue taking the antacids to control the excess stomach acid as well as the seizures. The original problem was not enough calcium to handle the healing of tissue and control of the seizure.

When the body gets into a state such as this, it may take several homeopathic remedies to get over the problem. Calcarea Carb. can treat the underlying calcium deficiency. Lycopodium can treat the problem with the extra acidity in the stomach. Silicea can set the acid level back to normal. All three of these remedies, taken one at a time and in the proper complementary order (as given here, all in the 30th potency) will usually work together to bring balance and normal function. **Do not take Silicea if you have implants or transplants in your body since Silicea may cause rejection or expulsion.**

15

The Role of Zinc in Weight Accumulation

Recent research suggests some people who suffer from anorexia are low in zinc. This initial problem may be the result of an inability of the body to absorb zinc from the diet or to process zinc into a usable energetic form. It is important to note that simply adding zinc to the diet cannot correct this underlying malfunction. No matter how much zinc is added, if the body cannot absorb and process it, the deficiency and the resulting anorexia will continue. It is the zinc deficiency that suppresses the appetite and, therefore, it is the zinc deficiency which must be corrected, homeopathically, to eliminate the anorexic behavior.

One day, a woman came to me with an anorexia-type problem, complaining that she wasn't able to eat. Food was repulsive, she had no appetite, and she was fearful that the battle with food was becoming serious. I suggested she try a dose of homeopathically potentized zinc, Zincum Metalicum. She took a 6X potency for a week. A month or so later she came to see me again for a different problem. I asked her how her anorexia was and she told me the problem had completely disappeared. Her appetite had returned and she had gained a few pounds. She was stunned to realize she had completely forgotten that the symptoms had ever been a problem at all.

• Zinc and Overeating

Let's take this discussion one step further. If an imbalance caused by the body's inability to absorb zinc can create anorexia as the result of a zinc deficiency, it is equally probable that the inability of the body to eliminate zinc would manifest as a weight related problem. In the case of a deficiency, you have anorexia or food avoidance and resulting weight loss. In the case of zinc overload, you have compulsive overeating with the resultant weight gain.

Several years ago, a throat lozenge appeared on the market in which a preparation of zinc was used to help the user get over the common symptoms of a cold. It was so effective and popular many companies jumped on the bandwagon and started marketing lozenges with zinc. What was misunderstood was that the first product on the market used homeopathically potentized zinc, which allowed the body to use zinc to boost the immune system without causing zinc accumulation. Many people who did not understand the difference, who used these later zinc lozenges, have found their lymphatic systems clogged, a reduction in immune response and their weight begin to rise inexplicably. This is all due to zinc accumulation where the body is unable to get rid of the excess mineral.

Specialists agree that one of the problems creating overweight conditions in today's population is the over consumption of "fast food". This food can come from "fast food" restaurants, food delivery services, take-out foods such as pizza and pre-processed food consumed in the home. Although the "high fat, low-fiber content" of such foods is a culprit in weight gain, there are other more basic problems related to this source of nutrition. The cans used for storing processed foods have high levels of zinc because the solder used in making the can is high in zinc. People may be getting an excess of zinc from the sauces on pizza, the condiments on burgers, and components of salad bars such as beans and olives--all foods that are stored and delivered in cans.

Additional sources for excess zinc in today's diet also stem from the belief that all supplements must contain "balanced nutrients" which are at levels often far exceeding the recommended daily allowance. The overwhelming belief that everyone must take daily supplements in order to avoid vitamin deficiencies and suffer ill health as a result of those deficiencies contributes to the zinc overload in people with this defect.

The diet is not the only source of zinc in today's lifestyle. Zinc oxide is often used as a preventative and treatment for diaper rash, eczema, psoriasis, sunburn and other skin aliments. Many forms of zinc are commonly found in products such as sun blocks, make-up, and as an all-natural coloring agent in consumable substances, all of which contribute to the zinc overload suffered by many people. The presence of zinc in all of these products is not a bad thing, since zinc is a necessary nutrient. What becomes a problem is the body's inability to eliminate excess zinc that is not needed. The question of why some bodies forget how to process and eliminate zinc properly is somehow related to the issue of calcium absorption deficiency. The two problems go hand in hand, but why this is so is not yet clear.

• Problems with Zinc

As zinc accumulates in overload, it becomes toxic to the body. If the body cannot eliminate the excessive, it must compensate by increasing the appetite and lowering the metabolism, thereby, increasing body weight. This increase in body weight serves to dilute the excess zinc with an increase in body mass. This increase of body mass is what the medical community attempts to address as a weight problem.

Unfortunately, as the person eats more food, more and

more zinc is also absorbed. As the person diets to "lose weight", they increase the concentration of zinc in their system due to zinc being liberated from the fat, causing the body to crave food to "fix" the concentration problem--regaining any weight lost to again create body mass and dilute the overload of zinc.

This syndrome, so common in today's world, has its own name, "Yo-Yo dieting". It is now considered a major problem, yet the allopathic medical community still has no adequate means to address it. The homeopathic system, on the other hand, has several techniques which address the original malfunction. One technique is to get rid of the excess zinc and solve the problems associated with zinc overload.

• Draining the Zinc

In Chapter 9 there is a discussion of chord potencies and how multiple potencies fall out of the body, draining the remedy along with the excess substance from which the remedy originated. This concept is critical in addressing issues such as zinc deficiency and overload. By using the correct potencies of precise remedies in specifically designed programs dictated by the symptoms and needs of each individual, it is possible to correct the underlying cause of the weight gain. By taking the proper remedies, the body will not only drain out the excess zinc, but also correct the mal-absorption problem. When this occurs, the individual cells of the body will absorb zinc properly as a nutrient, stop the excess storage of zinc and allow the body to get rid of excess bulk.

• Eliminating Toxins

Homeopathic remedies may, in many people, have an immediate impact in the reduction of an individual's weight--often beginning with the very first remedies. What is more likely, however, is that the changes the remedies make in mineral absorption and shifts in biochemistry will enable other weight control programs to work effectively, thereby, allowing people to obtain and maintain normal, optimum weight levels without suffering the "Yo-Yo" syndrome.

The problem with conventional weight loss programs is that they cause the release of toxins and other substances previously stored in fat which cannot be eliminated from the body. As the levels of these substances increase and the body again becomes overloaded, override mechanisms kick in, the appetite increases and the person starts to gain back weight as the body again attempts to neutralize the excess levels.

Homeopathic remedies used for weight control have subtle but definite effects. In one case, by balancing zinc, the client reported a steady decrease in appetite, loss of the fear of hunger, the ability to be "choosy" about food rather than simply consuming anything presented--as well as the ability to leave food on the plate after reaching a point of satisfaction. This client remarked that for the first time food was a choice and not simply a need.

In another case, also after balancing zinc, the client reported that the feeling of an intense need for food had diminished. This client also reported that this intense need for food was unrelated to any feeling of hunger, but simply occurred without any known reason.

Other changes reported include the loss of fear of physical activity and a corresponding increase in the desire for and pleasure in physical activity. One client reported that they couldn't remember a time in their life they didn't dread the idea of exercising, and found that they actually enjoyed the feeling of using the body after balancing zinc.

Still another client, after homeopathic treatment, reported not only a decrease in appetite along with a decrease in food consumption, but also a new feeling of mental clarity. This client had reported that when asked by a prior therapist, "what do you think about while you are eating?" She had realized that food and anger were so completely linked that it was impossible for her to eat without getting anger, or to get angry without eating. After using the appropriate remedy, she reported a definite release of the anger associated with eating and stated that for the first time since she could remember, she could sit and eat food and simply enjoy the experience. She also reported that when she became upset or angry she no longer found herself compulsively eating.

It is important to note that the mental changes associated with the homeopathic treatment of zinc accumulation occur because higher level potencies of homeopathic remedies act in the upper energy levels. In the case of zinc drainage, the 30th potency is acting on higher energy levels to drain excess zinc from brain tissue where it can accumulate as a pollutant and clog mental function activity and cause cloudy thinking. The drainage of excess zinc from the mental realms often results in the correct usage of zinc for mental function and a sensation of fog lifting from mental processes and new understanding of old thinking patterns.

• One Caution

The caution which one needs to observe when using homeopathic remedies to correct a weight control problem comes from a side effect related to the decreased consumption of food. As the appetite decreases, the amount of food being consumed also decreases, which decreases the amount of water and other fluids one takes in. Food is a major source of fluid for the body. One must be aware of the possibility of temporary slight dehydration as a result of the decrease in food. It is important to compensate by increasing the amount of fluids consumed, particularly at the beginning of a program. Because of the balancing action of homeopathic remedies, the likelihood that this problem will occur is very slight. If it does occur, it is normally very short lived and seldom presents any real problems.

Remember to use normal caution when doing exercise, participating in strenuous activity or simply conducting normal activity in hot weather. Remember, you must compensate with extra fluids for the loss of fluids from the food you are not eating or to replace fluids you lose through sweating.

When using zinc drainage remedies, it is not unusual to experience a temporary soreness and swelling in lymph glands throughout the body, particularly if you have been using zinc lozenges or taking zinc as a supplement. This is due to the fact that zinc accumulates in the glands, including salivary and prostate. When using the drainage remedy system, these glands will purge their accumulated zinc, causing soreness and swelling. After the initial purging, one may actually begin to feel proper lymph response when the immune system is fighting off an infection or an invading virus.

Another common sign of zinc accumulation is pain in the heels of the feet when stepping or walking. If the drainage of zinc causes a relief of just such a pain for you, the return of this pain would signal a new accumulation of zinc and a need to repeat the zinc drainage remedies.

The regime of how to use the remedies for zinc drainage appears in Chapter 16.

16

The Remedy Regime

What follows in this chapter is a regiment of remedies that benefits everyone. Some will see more results than others depending on their individuality, but in general, everyone benefits.

All of us alive in the world today have lost calcium through ageing, harmful environmental exposure, stress, physical trauma, errors in diet, or because we came into the world deficient due to our immigrant heritage. Restoring calcium improves the body's ability to heal injury, maintain immunity, stop recurring infections and stabilize weight. As I just said, we can all benefit.

Just remember, we are changing the way the body functions, permanently, without pain or mental effort. This change takes time, **but what else are you going to do the rest**

of your life. If you start this program now, in a year you will be an entirely different person. If you never start this program because it seems too complicated, too expensive, too long or too slow, where will you be in a year? You will still be calcium deficient, zinc overloaded, emotionally blocked and unable to lose weight. **What have you got to loss?**—except hidden weaknesses, excess weight, emotional baggage and nutrient deficiency. **What have you got to gain?**—your good health-- plus a whole new sense of well-being and mental clarity.

Not only can you stabilize your weight, make dieting more effective and feel better overall, you could also lose depression, fear, resentment, cravings and compulsive eating behavior.

• The First Stage

What follows is the schedule for making permanent changes. This remedy schedule may only need to be done once in a lifetime, or tuned up after a few years if there is injury, surgery, or extreme emotional shock, or if a person uses stimulants to lose weight or habitually drinks energy or workout drinks that contain ginseng or other herbal stimulants. The habitual use of these stimulants will shut down receptor sites on cells shutting off absorption of calcium and nutrients. This practice will always result in weight gain and calcium absorption deficiency.

If a new problem with calcium absorption arises, a person can repeat the remedies if they again feel themselves developing symptoms such as recurring infection, sweet or salt craving, or high stomach acidity.

All of these remedies are taken alone, only that remedy, taken for a period of only three days. Whether it is 30x or 30c does not matter, even if you follow a 30c with a 30x remedy, the distinction between the two dilution systems does not matter in the way a 30th potency works. What matters is that it was diluted 30 times, not which scale was used in the process (turn to Chapter 6 to review this concept if you need to).

In order to use a 30th potency one must purchase a 30th potency. Adding up potencies numbers and taking more than one potency at a time will result in drainage, which is not what we are working on.

Due to the compatibility rules of homeopathy and the relationship of remedies to each other, these remedies must be taken in the order presented here. If they are not taken in order, their effectiveness may be compromised.

Many of these remedies act for a very long duration of time, some for up to 60 to 90 days after they are taken. It is for this reason they are done in a complementary order. The remedies must be allowed to continue to work in conjunction with each other in a beneficial way. An individual will not be harmed by doing them out of order, but one can ruin the effectiveness of the remedy and increase the possibility of aggravations.

The remedies absorb through an energy portal under the tongue, not into the blood stream as previously thought. In order for this absorption to take place, there must be no food particles in the mouth. Before taking a remedy, be sure there has been nothing in the mouth, including water, for 15 minutes before putting the remedy under the tongue. Wait another 15 minutes after taking the remedy before allowing anything in the mouth. Put something in the mouth to close the portal and separate remedies from each other if taking more than one remedy in a day. This can be done with as little as a sip of water.

A dose is usually 4 pellets. The alcohol used to potentize the remedy is put on sugar pellets for easy use. A dose of 4 pellets makes a good coating under the tongue, however, if one is diabetic, or one wants to conserve the pellets for other people to use, it does not matter how many pellets are used for a dose. Remember, this is an energy impulse to energy bodies and not a material chemical based medicine. One pellet is a dose, as well as the whole bottle is a dose if taken at one time. Energy rules apply here, not the rules of substance building in the blood stream. If a child gets into the remedies and eats them, don't worry--even if they eat an entire bottle. Remember, to the body that does not need the remedy, the preparation is only sugar.

If the instruction is to "Wait a few days after taking a remedy", this means that one does not take another homeopathic remedy for three to four days, or longer, after finishing the three-day course of a 30th potency of a remedy. The time does not have to be specific or exact, use your own judgment as to how you feel or want to proceed. Just keep in mind that allowing more time for a remedy to work alone before another remedy is introduced is always a good thing with homeopathy. If you have to wait for a mail order deliver before you can begin your next remedy, just be assured time is good and no harm is done.

You may continue to take any pharmaceutical or herbal medicine that has been prescribed to you while you are taking a homeopathic remedy. Since pharmaceuticals and herbs are chemical based medicine and homeopathy is energy, the two forces never meet. In spite of what you may have heard from other homeopathic practitioners, there is no harm to the homeopathy in continuing with your regular medication. You will need to ask your doctor about this regime if you are on many medications or suffer a serious illness.

Understand that if you do choose to follow this regime, it is of your own accord. I am imparting knowledge I have gained over many years of experience in the hope that others benefit from what I have learned, but I am not a medical doctor and I am not forcing anyone to do anything against their better judgment. I cannot be held responsible for any perceived harm that may result from the use of these remedies, nor for the lack of results,

since many factors undetectable and not related to homeopathy may be at cause.

Remember, homeopathic remedies are energy based and do not impact directly on the physical body. A homeopathic remedy cannot cause or aggravate a situation that is not already present. I am not responsible for the misunderstanding of these concepts if the previous chapters have not been read by the individual.

Check with your doctor before beginning a weight reduction program. This is good advice at any time, but particularly if one's physical state is less than good.

Do not choose homeopathy over the advice of your regular physician. Homeopathy does not replace the treatment your doctor may have already recommended, but homeopathy may be used as a complement to regular treatment if your doctor so agrees.

• Sodium and Calcium absorption:

Remember, each remedy is taken alone, for a period of three days only. After completion of the three days, go on to the next remedy. That means, Natrum Mur. 30th potency is taken alone, three times a day for a period of three days. At the completion of this three-day-period, go on to Calcarea Carb.

If for some reason, one does not complete the three day period because they forgot to continue to take doses, and there is a gap of more than 24 hours since the last dose, do not attempt to go back and make up the difference. Just continue to the next remedy. This is done because homeopathic remedies are an energy impulse to the energy bodies and follow different rules than material medicine. If an energy impulse has begun with a few doses and interrupted by a period of time, beginning the remedy again will cause a clash of energy impulses and antidote the effect of the remedy. If only one dose is missed, proceed with the remedy to complete the three-day-cycle.

• The Remedy Regime in Proper Order

Day 1, 2 and 3--Mark you Calendar
Natrum Mur.   30th potency, X or C (either one, it doesn't matter which), but 30 is essential

Take the remedy in a 4 pellet dose under the tongue, three times a day for three days. At the completion of this three-day-period, stop taking it and put it away. It is best to wait a few days and give it some time to work on its own. This can be 2 to 4 days depending on how you as an individual feel in regard to waiting. If you are anxious and want to go on, make it two days. If you are experiencing changes in the way you feel and think, wait 4 days before continuing on.

Day 4, 5 and 6 of remedy regime (not calendar days)
Calcarea Carb. 30

3 doses a day for three days only and wait a few days as above. This is calcium carbonate already converted to energy to open receptor sites on cells to accept the calcium molecule.

Day 7, 8 and 9
Lycopodium 30

3 doses a day for three days only and wait a few days. Lycopodium is a remedy from the plant kingdom that helps to hold the new receptor sites open to continue to absorb calcium.

Day 10,12 and 13
Sulphur 30

3 doses a day for three days only and wait a few days. This is elemental sulfur, a necessary nutrient that is often lacking where calcium absorption is low. This remedy allows sulfur to be absorbed into cells along with calcium.

Calc. Phos. 6X

3 doses a day for a period of at least a month. This 6X potency works on the innermost energy bodies ensuring continued calcium absorption into deep internal layers of the body.

1	2	3	4	5	6	7
Natrum Mur. 3 x Today	Natrum Mur. 3 x Today	Natrum Mur. 3 x Today		*wait* →		
8 Calcarea Carb. 3x today	**9** Calcarea Carb. 3x today	**10** Calcarea Carb. 3x today	**11**	**12** *wait* →	**13**	**14**
15 Lycopodium 3x today	**16** Lycopodium 3x today	**17** Lycopodium 3x today	**18**	**19** *wait* →	**20**	**21**
22 Sulphur 3x today	**23** Sulphur 3x today	**24** Sulphur 3x today	**25**	**26** *wait* →	**27**	**28**
29	**30** Calc. Phos. 6X Every day for a month	**31**				

If you are very calcium deficient, you may want to continue to take Calc. Phos. 6X for many months, or as long as you feel changes occurring in muscle tone.

Beginning a calcium supplement as you begin the Calc. Phos. 6X is appropriate. Any supplement product made by any reputable company in a dosage of 500mg to 1000mg taken once a day is fine. Do not overdose on calcium by taking 2000mg. Overdosing is not going to help. Take the calcium with food, since it needs stomach acid to break it down into useable components. Choose a supplement that also contains magnesium--magnesium and calcium are always absorbed together. Boron or Vitamin D included in the calcium supplement is okay, but it is best to avoid a product that includes zinc since zinc can accumulate in tissue and cause toxicity.

Calcarea homeopathic remedies begin absorption of calcium into the cells, but do not provide the nutrient. Supplementation provides the nutrient, but without the absorption signal from the homeopathic remedy, calcium does not go into the cells. Both forms of calcium are necessary. As long as you are taking a calcium supplement, you should take at least one dose a day of Calc. Phos. 6X, or a related calcarea remedy (such as Calc. Sulph. 6X or Calc. Fluor. 6X). This is easily achieved by taking one dose of Calc. Phos.6X as you lay down to sleep at night. This dose will help improve the quality of sleep.

Add Mag. Phos. 6X during the day in a two pellet dose from time to time. This will ensure that magnesium is absorbed correctly along with the calcium. If magnesium is not being absorbed correctly, one may experience muscle cramping, stiffness in the lower legs and a return of migraine headaches.

Also, a one month course of Natrum Mur. 6X taken during the day on the same day as a bedtime dose of Calc. Phos. 6X will help a person get over the sodium deficiency associated with emotional trauma by clearing the emotional upset from the deepest energy bodies. This will help bring about mental clarity and increase mental function.

The 6X potency is so physical in its action one does not have to worry about restarted at any time after a period of stopping it for another remedy, or even if one forgets to take a 6X potency remedy for a few days. In other words, a 6X or 6C potency can be started and stopped or interrupted at any time with impunity.

Some people will begin to lose weight at this time merely by causing calcium absorption. Others will begin to experience a reduction in inches without weight loss as their body takes on moisture and density. For many, weight lose will begin because the person will feel more inclined to move around and become more active. For those who do not have weight to lose, immunity and cell repair capabilities will improve. Mood and muscle tone will improve as well. Women will see a much more dramatic change than men. However, everyone who is overweight will benefit.

• The Simple Regime

If your lifestyle or your skepticism leaves you unsure or unable to follow the complete remedy regime, you can achieve the same benefit by using only three remedies. It will take a longer period of time to get the full benefit, but it will work.

Start with a daily dose of Natrum Mur. 6X in the morning hours of your day. This dose insures the body is absorbing sodium correctly and moisturizing the bones in order to take on new calcium and density. Next, a daily dose of Mag. Phos. 6X in the afternoon hours. This dose will insure the body is absorbing magnesium which goes hand in hand with calcium. Lack of magnesium can lead to migraine headaches and muscle stiffness. Finally, a daily dose of Calc. Phos. 6X at the time you are going to bed will make sure the body is absorbing calcium correctly. This is good to take at night because calcium calms the nervous system and sleep improves. The effect is similar to warm milk or ice cream before bed.

These three remedies can be taken in doses of one to two pellets everyday, all three at separate times on each day, along with a mild calcium supplement that includes magnesium. Try to find one without zinc. If you continue this simple regime for up to a year, you will see the same benefits as taking the complete program in 30th potencies. The deficiencies will take longer to resolve and changes in the body will come more slowly--but it will work.

• Second Stage--Toxin Drainage

It is now time to drain zinc, and by the way, other heavy metal toxins will drain with the zinc. These may include lead, aluminum and mercury.

Remember, a chord is three potencies taken at the same time, in the same mouthful, once a day for 5 days. If you try to take more than this, aggravations may occur, such as headache or stomach ache. If you have not yet read what a chord potency is, please turn to chapter 9 and read the action of the multiple potency chord doses.

You will need to purchase three different potencies of **Zincum Metallicum (Zincum Met.)** The first one will be a 30th potency, 30X or 30C, either one is fine. The second one is a potency in the teens, either a 12th potency or a 15th potency. It does not matter if it is a 12X or a 12C. The difference between X and C potencies is not a difference that matters with this schedule. Finally, the third one is a low potency, either a 3X or a 6X. If you can find only a 6C, that is fine, the distinction does not matter, but these low potency numbers are usually made in X's. **The dose is one pellet from each of the three bottles (one pellet of each of the three potencies—a 30th, a 12th and a 6X for example), a total of 3 pellets, taken all together in the same mouthful, only once a day for a total of 5 days.**

This Chord potency is taken only once a day, therefore, it can be done on the days that you are doing Calc. Phos. 6X in three potencies a day (or while taking the three remedies of the simple regime). In other words, after you have finished the first 4 remedies taken in 30th potencies, begin taking your daily dose of the Zincum Met. Chord, and take your 3 doses of Calc. Phos. 6X on the same day. Eat or drink something after the doses of the chord remedies and before the Calc. Phos. 6X dose in order to shut the portal so the next dose goes through separately.

Do not overdue the use of the zinc drainage chord. This remedy regime should only be repeated if one loses a lot of weight and the heels become sore from zinc being liberated from fat tissue. Otherwise, once a year is often enough. Using these drainage remedies too often may result in drainage of metals used by the body as nutrients.

• Old Infections Aggravate

After a person has taken the calcium absorption remedies and has been taking calcium supplements for a while, it is not unusual for that person to feel pain and old symptoms in areas of the body where there had been infection in the past. I am telling you this so you will be prepared when it happens.

A client called just the other day to say she was having chills and a feverish feeling accompanied by tightness in the chest. The symptoms disappeared after twelve hours or so and she was fine, but she was concerned as to why it had happened. I told her the absorption of calcium into the cells where old infection occurred is the effect of the immune system getting rid of the remnants of the infection once and for all. She confirmed she had had a life-long problem with upper-respiratory infections. I have seen this in many of my clients using this regime.

My experience has been very interesting. In the first few months of taking calcium supplements along with a dose of Calc. Phos. 6X everyday, all the places where I had had root canal work aggravated and became sore. The soreness went away within 24 hours but returned about two weeks later for a quick rebound, never to return again. I had thought those places had been cleared up with antibiotics, but apparently something remains to be cleared on the cellular level when the immune system can handle it with the increased calcium.

I had an even more interesting experience with kidney pain. I have had kidney infections since I was a child of 3 years old. One day, about eight months after I had started the calcium supplement regime, I woke up in the morning with severe back pain. I knew it was my kidneys and it felt as if the same old infection had come back. I was giving my son a graduation party that day so I didn't stop to go to the doctor, but I was in pain the entire day. By evening I was running a fever and wondered if I would have to see a doctor the following day. Late in the evening the fever started to drop. I went to bed, hoping I wouldn't get worse during the night, but vowing to see a doctor if I did. I woke the next morning feeling fine with no pain and no fever. Two weeks later there was a minor recurrence of the pain, which went away the same day. Now I feel perfectly healthy and for the first time in my life, at least since I was three years old, I do not feel the need to pamper myself just in case fatigue or over exertion might lead to an infection.

The aggravation of old infections can be painful and frightening. If these aggravations are caused by the infusion of calcium into tissue where infection has occurred in the past, it will be temporary. **<u>However, do not hesitate to see a doctor if the pain is severe, accompanied by fever, or lasts for more than 24 hours.</u>**

If what you are feeling is a new infection and not an aggravation, the symptoms will get worse and will not subside in a reasonable amount of time. Definitely see a doctor if this is the case. Untreated infection can lead to permanent damage.

• Continue Calcium

After the calcium absorption regime, the sodium balancing regime and the zinc drainage regime, it is important to return to a daily calcium absorption regime for at least several months.

During this time, perhaps on alternating months, switch to other calcium related remedies in 6X potencies such as Calc. Sulph., Calc. Fluorica and Natrum Carb. This will ensure that you are absorbing calcium into every form of tissue in the body. For example, one month, use Calc. Phos.6X. In the next month switch to Calc. Fluor. 6X and continue until the bottle is finished. When you go to buy a new bottle, get Nat. Carb. 6X and take it until you finish the bottle. The Calc. Fluor. strengthens connective tissue and blood vessels, Calc. Sulph. strengthens skin tissues and the Nat. Carb. is a component of tissues influenced by both sodium and calcium, which include the brain and internal organs. All are beneficial in restoring and maintaining good health. And don't forget Mag. Phos. 6X for a week or so from time to time.

It is a good idea to take small amounts of Vitamin C, 250 to 500 mg a day, to improve the integrity of blood vessels and muscle tone in conjunction with the calcium absorption regime. Vitamin C will help the body feel satisfied and allow for less food consumption. Large amounts of Vitamin C are usually thrown out of the body causing deficiency. Large doses of Vitamin C scour the inside of blood vessels and can be cleansing if this action is needed for a short time. However, continuing to take large doses can actually cause cuts and tears in the blood vessels. Small amounts work best for long term nutritional needs and improving the integrity of blood vessels.

Also, adding Bilberry extract as a dietary supplement will improve eyesight. As all other blood vessels and tissues in the body are strengthening and building tone, the Bilberry herb in capsule form will help improve the function of the eyes by providing the micro nutrients necessary for those specialized structures.

I do not agree with the idea that a daily multi-vitamin supplement is necessary for good health. Most of what the body needs will be derived from the nutrients mentioned already. Many vitamins contain too many elements in potencies too high to be good on an ongoing basis. Taking a multi-vitamin from time to time is good just to make sure everything the body needs is made available; say one or two capsules a week on alternate days. I tend to take a multi-vitamin once a week for a few weeks a year.

The problem with lots of excess nutrients is that many can accumulate in tissue as a waste product because the body had no place to put it, or force the body to constantly eliminate, causing stress. The same is true for herbal supplements. The overuse of herbal supplements can be very difficult for the body, causing the body to react to a constant stimulation that is not necessary. Remember, if an herb had not become a food in the indigenous culture from which it originated, it cannot be taken without some sort of side effect, even if that is a long term effect that seems remote for years. Somewhere down the road there will be problem.

• Dietary Overload

The need of a calcium deficient body to obtain the nutrient it cannot absorb leads to the situation where the person is not able to distinguish between what is beneficial to good health and proper nutrition and what is desired to be eaten. These are the people who will only stop eating when the belt is tight and no more food will fit in the stomach. This situation leads to the need to control diet by extraordinary means such as the fad diets that restrict certain food groups. This is the external attempt to control eating because the natural controls the body would impose in the state of proper balance are not available to the person who experiences this problem.

As the body becomes balanced with proper nutrients, the ability to control eating will become a natural process. When this occurs, the need for fad dieting will be eliminated and person will feel the proper responses to hunger and satiation. At that time, it will be easy to adhere to a routine that allows for proper weight balance. Proper weight balance is the situation where the person is neither too thin nor burdened with excess weight.

The best diet to achieve the proper weight balance is to eat several small meals a day of foods from all the food groups. Eating whatever one desires, in small amounts, finishing at the first feeling of fullness, not when the belt is as tight as possible, is probably the best strategy. Knowing that one will not be able to over eat should lead one to think and plan the meals, choosing nutritious foods, not just whatever is around as may have been the habit in the past. Do not restrict or eliminate any one food group, and that includes dessert, but everything should be taken in very small amounts.

The diets that restrict a particular type of food can lead to cravings, causing overeating. If one is aware of how the body feels and what it really desires, it becomes easy to eat what is needed and desired for proper nutrition.

I cannot tell you how many times I have heard people on sugar restricted diets for yeast reduction or weight control talk about not being able to stop themselves from falling into a sugar binge. Guilt and self-loathing followed rapidly. The person of course was unaware the body craved the sugar because it had to have it for proper function.

Sugar is a nutrient needed for the natural lubrication on the internal organs so they do not stick together when we move. Sugar is also an important nutrient for many functions in the body, including brain activity and information processing. The body cannot function without a certain amount of sugar.

The body must have carbohydrates. Low carbohydrate/ high protein diets can only be done for a short period of time before serious carbohydrate deficiency problems begin. These include bloating, fluid retention, starvation responses from the liver and lowered brain function.

Low fat diets only lead to the body craving fat and

rebounding with increased weight gain to compensate. The function and health of nerve tissue is dependent on fat in the diet. The human body cannot survive without fat. Those who have been on low fat diets for a long time may experience chronic nerve pain, sciatic pain, or nerve disorders with symptoms resembling those of Parkinson's Disease. Many people on low fat diets have experienced gall bladder problems due to the back up of bile in the gall bladder because of the decrease in bile secretions when there is little fat in the diet.

It is best to eat very small meals, up to five times a day, from every food group in order to include all nutrients. Decreasing calorie intake slowly to a point where pounds can be lost is a good idea in order to avoid putting the liver in survival mode by starting a diet abruptly.

Let us not forget, overeating will cause weight gain no matter what we do to diet. Often, the balance between overeating and good nutrition is difficult to determine. As cells become properly nourished, satiation responses should become normal, eliminating the need to control the impulse to overeat. However, it will still be necessary to increase physical activity and control calorie intake in order to lose large amounts of weight.

17

Metabolic Syndrome

Are you a victim of weight-loss diet overexposure? Have you been on a diet your entire life? Have you used stimulants to raise your metabolism and diet drinks to cut calories? Have you tried every diet that was ever invented and gained more weight after every one? Are you suffering from an allergy to dieting? In other words, are you unable to stick to a diet because your body reacts badly every time you try. Are you truely unable to lose weight? Skinny heiresses seem to know how not to get into this situation. What do they know we don't?

All of these attempts to lose wieght produce a compensation illness as well as an inappropriate learning disease. Anytime the body is forced to do something against its nature, a compensation response will occur, leading to a deeper and deeper problem. An inappropriate learning disease is created as the body continues to respond to what it has learned even after of the chemical is removed. Restoring the body's natural responses is not easy to do, but always preferable to using another substance to force the body to shut off natural function in order to control the newer learned response.

• Syndrome X

Metabolic Syndrome or Syndrome X is a condition in which the body becomes resistant to insulin. The insulin resistant person is described as pre-diabetic and in danger of developing diabetes type 2. Common signs are a waistline over 35 inches in women/40 inches in men, a fasting blood sugar level over 100mg/100mL and a very difficult time when trying to lose weight. This situation arises as insulin receptor sites on individual cells that are supposed to take in nutrients from the blood stop functioning. The number of functioning receptor sites become reduced in number. The number of functioning receptor sites is far less than normal and glucose cannot be absorbed into cells correctly due to this deficiency in available working sites. Cells starve for the needed glucose and the individual feels weak from the deprivation. The blood stream remains high in glucose concentration, the body reads that the blood sugar is high and releases more insulin; resulting in the body tissues becoming allergic to the over abundance of insulin in the blood. During this over-release of insulin into the blood, glucose is stored quickly in the abdominal area to get it out of the blood stream since it didn't go into cells as it should have; resulting in weight gain in the middle of the body and storage of glucose in areas where it shouldn't be stored, such as the liver, internal organs and the skin.

The appetite remains high because the cells are still unfed. Attempts to lose weight by skipping meals are undermined by the liver, which throws out excess glucose to feed the cells because the liver perceives that starvation is the reason for all of this chaos. The cells use the glucose delivered by the liver instead of metabolizing it from stored fat. Eventually, the body shuts down insulin production, resulting in diabetes.

• What has started all of this?

In my opinion, there are basically three factors that have caused this insulin resistance problem.

The first factor is the calcium deficiency situation described earlier in the book. Most people who fall into the insulin resistance category will have started life as calcium deficient or became that way after surgery, injury or intense emotional upset. For some reason, cells stopped absorbing calcium, which led to lower than normal metabolism, poor muscle tone and improper immune response. In this situation, fat cells have a tendency to be larger than normal. The result is an overweight sedentary person who is prone to trying anything to lose weight.

The second factor is the use of stimulants to aid weight loss. All of us diet junkies have used these products at one time or another. These stimulants include amphetamines, ephedrine, ginseng, Fen®Phen®, excessive caffeine products; any product taken as a drug or dietary supplement that temporarily increases body metabolism and supposedly burns fat. This includes those new energy drinks that have become so popular.

The problem is that stimulants do over-stimulate the individual cells of the body. For a time, this causes the cells to use more glucose and nutrients to keep up, which raises the metabolism level of the individual resulting in weight loss. After some time, the cells give up and can no longer tolerate all of this stimulation; they close off receptor sites in order to protect themselves from further stimulation (a compensation response). The result is that the product no longer works, working receptor sites are reduced, glucose does not go into the cells properly because receptor sites do not return to normal after the stimulant is stopped (inappropriate learning) and the person regains the weight. Also, more weight is gained because now the cells will not take in the amount of glucose they did before the product was taken. The cells fail to be nourished and calories consumed by the individual are stored instead of used.

A high level of emotional upset will cause the same response. The cells can not tolerate the constant presence of stimulating chemicals present in the blood due to emotional stress over a period of time or in recurring patterns and the cells shut down receptor sites.

These two situations are aggravating causes of calcium deficiency. If the person was not calcium deficient before taking the stimulant or experiencing the emotion, they will become so after. The receptor sites that shut down to prevent the excess stimulation from entering the cells also stop calcium from entering the cells. It takes time to develop, but all the symptoms of calcium deprivation described earlier will develop. This includes poor muscle tone and a lowered ability to burn calories through exercise. The solution is the calcium absorption regime described in Chapter 16.

The third factor in this insulin resistance problem is the use of diet drinks. Most people who have dieted frequently throughout their lifetime have used diet drinks during most of that time. As a person drinks a drink with artificial dietary sweeteners, the sweet taste sends signals to the brain and the body that sugar is forthcoming. The body releases sugar-controlling insulin, but no sugar appears in the blood stream. However, the tissues have to deal with the excess insulin since there was no sugar to be broken down, causing the tissue to become allergic and resistant to the presence of excess insulin and more receptor sites shut down to prevent insulin from entering the cells without glucose. Because of the excess insulin in the blood stream, the person becomes hungry and begins to eat. Since the blood stream is high in insulin concentration that is not going into cells, the next calories consumed are stored in the abdominal area.

• Arrest the Problem

Stop drinking diet sodas and saccharine flavored drinks, or use them only while eating a meal. Skinny heiresses don't drink diet drinks, give them up now.

Don't use any stimulate to help in weight loss—including energy drinks. Coffee does not seem to affect the receptor sites if the amount of coffee consumed on a daily basis is less than 3 to 4 cups, or the equivalent consumed throughout the day. Avoid putting saccharine in your coffee.

Do the remedy regime in Chapter 16. The use of the calcium absorption remedies opens up new receptor sites in the cells to receive calcium, which remain open to receive glucose from insulin, thereby increasing nutrient absorption into cells dramatically. (more remedies to solve this problem will be explained in a forthcoming publication)

• Diet Virgins

If you are a diet virgin, a person who has never really dieted before, you are unlikely to have a problem with insulin resistance unless you have been under stress for a long period of time, have had trouble sleeping for an extended period, or have suffered a major emotional event.

A diet virgin is a person who has not created the compensation response in the body that leads to a shut down of receptor sites. It is easy for a diet virgin to lose weight, the body does not yet know what is to come. This person can use any diet and lose weight. It is usually a diet virgin who becomes the poster child for a new diet aid product as it hits the market; you know them, the person who lost a lot of weight without any problem and kept it off. We were all able to do that in the beginning.

However, as time, stress, emotion and failed diets jade the body against dieting and increases insulin resistance, no diet will work. Keep this in mind when you hear those ads for the next great diet plan or product.

What is never really addressed is that most of us are not diet virgins and do not lose weight on any of these products, but the manufacturers want us to think we can and spend our money. Most of us are diet junkies and none of these diets or products work for us in actually creating weight loss.

If you are a diet junkie, you may have developed problems with the following diets.

• Low Fat Diets

Many people who have lost a lot of weight on a low fat diet program have experienced a problem with the gall bladder. Many of these people have actually had their gall bladder surgically removed because of the pain and problems that developed while on this diet.

The problem is that a low-fat diet can cause bile to back up in the gall bladder because the lack of fat in the diet reduces bile secretions.

If you are one of the people who has tried a low-fat diet, and you still have your gall bladder, but have some minor pain in the region, there is help. Gall bladder pain in its mildest form will be experienced as a pain or uncomfortable feeling under the right scapular bone, or the right shoulder blade. Sometimes this pain is so mild the person will only describe it as a tired feeling and attribute it to fatigue. However, it is most often mild radiated pain from the gall bladder. More severe pain will be actual pain on the right side of the abdomen above or at the waist—not to be confused with pain of the appendix in the low right abdomen.

If this pain is severe, do not hesitate to see a doctor and expect the surgical removal of the gall bladder. If this problem continues for too long untreated, the tissue of the gall bladder can die, causing serious complications. The homeopathic remedy suggested here is for reversal of a mild problem at a point at which the problem can be reversed by the body. The pop artist Andy Warhol actually lost his life due to neglected gall bladder disease. This is not a condition to take lightly.

If your discomfort is mild and you want to try to reverse the condition, the remedy is Cinchona Officinalis (common name is China, or Peruvian Bark) in a 30, X or C potency, taken three times a day for 3 days only. This is followed with the mother tincture of Chelidonium Majus, (a liquid herbal tincture potentized in a 1X), taken by adding several drops of the liquid to a small amount of water and swallowed into the stomach two to three times a day for a period of one month. This regime can put the gall bladder in order and reset the survival mode of the liver that began with deprivation during dieting.

Other remedies that help the gall bladder heal after these first two remedies are Aurum Met. 6X and Carbo Veg. 6X, taken in alternating doses through the day, one to two doses of one to two pellets each remedy, each day for a period of about a month.

• The High Fat--low Carb Diet

The elimination of carbohydrates from the diet is a very dangerous prospect. The compensation symptoms the body will produce could include bloating, constipation, water retention, mental fogginess, kidney pain and possibly kidney stones. Carbohydrates are absolutely necessity for normal function of the body and the brain. The reduction of carbohydrates in the diet may be okay for a short period of time, and may actually produce weight loss, but long term use of this diet can be a problem. Any weight lost is usually regained quickly.

The kidneys suffer greatly during this diet because the kidneys became responsible for eliminating the by-products of protein metabolism which are very harsh and taxing to the tiny filtration structures in the kidneys. The high protein aspect can also inhibit calcium absorption causing stones to form in the kidneys. Ask any veterinarian about the problems that cats face more often than any other problem. Because cats are carnivorous by nature and normally eat a diet high in protein, the major challenge to cat health is kidney failure.

The remedy to help relieve stress to the kidneys is Lycopodium, 30th potency, three times a day for three days, followed by Kali Phos. 6X for a month after. This is general advice to eliminate any problem that may have arisen, even problems that you are not aware of, in order to eliminate the stress low-carb dieting may have caused to your system. The calcarea remedy of the Chapter 16 regime will also help eliminate the excess calcium associated with the possible formation of kidney stones.

Again, if the problem is severe and there is pain, do not hesitate to see a doctor for the surgical removal of kidney stones. This can be a life-threatening situation and should not be ignored.

• Stomach Surgery

Those who have gone through the surgical procedure to staple the stomach and eliminate the capacity for large amounts of food in order to correct morbid obesity may find that after some time the weight starts to return. This is because the underlying problem of calcium mal-absorption and insulin resistance that caused the problem in the first place has not been taken care of and the cells of the body are still unable to find satiation. The calcium absorption regime of Chapter 16 will help balance the problem. Zinc drainage will help eliminate excess zinc that will have been liberated through fat loss and stop the body's need to dilute the zinc concentration with new weight gain.

• Vegetarianism

Vegetarian diets, which are usually very low in fat can be a problem for the body also. Most people on vegetarian diets will have problems healing after injury, injure the body more frequently due to tissue weakness and have very low resistance to disease. Most of this is due to the deficiency of amino acids, which are necessary nutrients found naturally in animal proteins. One meal of chicken a week would help greatly to relieve some of these symptoms.

So, basically, any diet that eliminates a particular food group is not good for the human body. In order to stay healthy, we cannot completely eliminate meat, carbohydrates, fat or sugars. In spite of best intentions or a desire to compensate kindness for cruelty to another living species, the reality is that human beings possess an animal body that is part of the food chain of this planet. Don't forget that plants are a living species also. We cannot go against our normal body need for proper nutrients as inherited from our development in a particular geographic area or lifestyle and remain healthy as individuals.

• Recognize the New You

It is often a problem that upon losing a lot of weight and beginning to look good, a person will look in the mirror one day and feel that they are not the same person as before and begin a campaign to regain the person they used to be. In order to stop this process and need to find the old person that has now been lost, a single dose of the homoeopathic potentized form of Valerian Root, Valeriana in a 1M or 1,000th potency will help the person recognize the new person they have become and feel comfortable in their new self image. This single dose can be repeated from time to time as weight is lost over a long period.

18

Finding the Holy Grail

The legends and quest stories surrounding the Holy Grail have captured Western imagination since The Middle Ages. The tradition of stories surrounding the search for the cup of Christ spans a range of over 800 years, from the Arthurian Legends to Indiana Jones.

Perhaps the Grail is—as it has come to be used in modern language--not an object, nor a person, but rather an ideal. Perhaps it is an inner knowing, an ability to understand the mysteries of life and the truths of nature. Perhaps it is an ideal attainable by ordinary men, indeed intended for use by mankind—and when it is found mankind will understand himself and his true relationship to God.

• What We Want from Life

Is it not true that everyone wants to be happy? When we are young, don't we expect that life will bring us good times and happy relationships? At least that is what we are led to believe should happen. Why is it not always the way we expect and want it to be? In our attempts to find happiness, we follow what the consumer driven authority of the society we live in dictates to us never realizing there are other ways to be. Malcontent occurs as what we were promised in our youth does not materialize as we were told it should. (Remember The Rembrandt's song at the beginning of the Television show "Friends". "No one told me it was going to be this way.")

Most people have lost the capacity to discern between the words of one who speaks with genuine authority and knowing and one who speaks with false or superficial knowledge. This is because most people do not listen with the intent to understand, which is mostly due to the inability of the brain to process information on a higher level. This is not the fault of the individual as many have been told. It is a malfunction in brain chemistry. I know because I have spent most of my life in the same situation. The good news is that there are remedies that can improve the thinking processes of everyone who uses them. I know because my thinking has changed.

The body that has been calcium deficient on physical levels will undoubtedly be lacking in other minerals necessary for higher mental functions as well. I have found this to be true in most cases and there is a solution. After doing the calcium absorption remedies and zinc drainage remedies already described in this book, it is time to do a few remedies to improve the ability of the brain to actually form new cells to receive information that will allow for higher functions of the mind. This ability is much more physical than many have been led to believe in the past.

After the completion of a few months of the remedy Calc. Phos. 6X, it is appropriate to take Thyroidium in a 6th potency, three times a day for the period of one month. After the completion of this month, one may notice a shift in understanding due to the opening of new areas of the brain to circulation and stabolize hormonal influence.

At this time, begin a process of infusing the mineral copper into the brain in order to form new brain cells that will be capable of carrying new information and form new thought patterns. This is done with very small amounts of copper as a supplement, no more than 30 micrograms a day is needed.

In addition to the supplement capsule of copper, Cuprum Met. in the 6th potency is taken to ensure absorption. This homeopathic form of copper is taken two to three times a day for a few weeks time. After a few weeks, stop both remedies. Allow the brain some time to create changes, and go back to these two forms of copper again for a short time a few months later.

Remember, only a minute amount is needed. Excess copper will not be beneficial. Have you ever experienced an itching sensation in the throat when eating melon or tomatoes? This is a sign your body was not absorbing copper as a nutrient correctly. If you go through a craving for tomatoes or melon after taking Cuprum Met., it is a sign your body has not been absorbing copper and wants you to eat it from a natural source. Indulge the craving.

• What would make us happy?

Maybe that illusive term "happiness" is in reality freedom. Freedom from the effects of past traumatic events on an individual's personal mindset.

Think of it. What if every human being alive today could be free from the fear created by improper subconscious decisions and biochemical imbalances and able to step out into the larger world created by correct understanding? Societies would evolve and happiness would be genuine.

Fear takes many forms. One form of fear is displayed by the person who stays in the job he hates, the town he grew up in, or the house she lived in for thirty years for fear of leaving the routine and trying something different. Most of these people are miserable and want more out of life, but are not aware of why they fail to try for more. (Arsenicum Album in a 30th potency is a remedy that helps eliminate this sort of fear. Caution: Read the entire book to understand how and why this remedy is used.)

Another form of fear is the paranoid fear that makes people push for control, feel the need to be in control at all times and become exhausted in the constant attempt to make sure they are in control. These are the people who appear powerful to the rest of us. In reality they are unapproachable, unlovable and unable to form lasting relationships. These people have to make sure no one comes close enough to cause them harm.

This type of paranoid fear is a reaction most often learned as a small child, usually before the individual was old enough to understand the manipulation of care giving adults. This fearful reaction is often seen in the person who was subjected to hospitalization as an infant. If an individual has suffered the trauma of injury, major surgery, major illness or long separation from the birth mother for any reason, it would be reasonable to expect that person to display some degree of fearful behavior.

These fear producing events are unavoidable. Of course it is far better the individual survives as a result of hospital care than not to be subjected to it. And yet it is easy to see how many individuals may well be affected by this type of fear, most of them unaware of the problem. (Kali Bromatum in a single 1M potency dose helps to clear this problem homeopathically).

Still another form of fear is actually physical. This form is the result of a frightening experience that has left the person dazed and confused with headaches, anxiety attacks and difficult or shallow breathing. This fear is the acute fear that makes the person's heart palpitate, his face turn red and makes him feel afraid of people, thunder, lightening, the nighttime, or a knock on the door.

This fear could have originated with a back injury, whiplash, spinal administered medication, or minor percussion blows to the spinal area. This is why I say this is a physical fear. It is actually the result of interruption in the flow of spinal fluid though the spinal column. The fluid around the brain is less than it should be and the person becomes fearful. I have seen this symptom in school children who carry large heavy backpacks to school allowing the bag to impact the spine while the child plays or runs. The result is night terrors, insomnia or a general fearfulness of anyone and anything.(The remedy is Aconitum Nap. taken in a 30th potency three times a day for three days—and only three days--to relieve the symptoms, followed with Natrum Mur. 6X for a month to put moisture back in the spinal column.)

• The Formation of Anger

What if a person were perfectly happy until something occurred in their life that made them feel worthless. This is the result of being shamed by the actions of another person trying to make himself appear powerful.

This sort of shaming can be perpetrated by a parent, a sibling, a classmate or a spouse. It can also be the result of crime victimization, but always the result is deep seated anger.

It is anger so deep a person feels pain because of it. It clouds their entire life and impacts every aspect of it. This pain can hurt so much the person doesn't want to be in the body. These are the people who either numb themselves with alcohol or drugs, or actually remove their soul from the physical body by disengaging the energy bodies.

This may sound strange, how can it be that a person disengages and floats out of the body? It is not a complete levitation out, but rather a blurring of the lines of connectedness, just enough disengagement to dull the sensations of pain, and the person in his conscious mind would be totally unaware this has occurred.

When this disconnectedness does occur, the person no longer feels hunger, fullness, physical pain, love or pleasure. These people are frequently overeaters because they have no idea when the body needs nourishment, when it has had too much or when it is suffering from the effects of over indulgence. These are also the people many others describe as "dead inside". They are the people who are unable to cry, feel sadness or express emotion. These people will also crave foods high in salt content, such as chips, pretzels or cheese snacks because sodium absorption has been interrupted by the emotion, which causes an entire complex of additional problems.

To clear the problem of anger, the homeopathic remedy is Alfalfa in a 30th potency, taken three times a day for three days only.

(To restart sodium absorption and relieve the craving that would have begun with grief, anger, or fear, the remedy is Natrum Mur. in a 6X potency for a few weeks.)

• The Effects of Grief

Consider how a person would feel if everything in their life were going great until suddenly something so profound happened they felt as though they could not continue and every day was the same as the day of the tragic event. This is what profound grief feels like. It is common for a person in this situation to feel they could no longer make progress or even advance to the next day. The early death of a loved one and an accident that takes a child are examples of events so traumatic as to create this sort of grief. Sometimes it does not have to be so devastating an event. Sometimes the loss of a job or a move to a new city will create this reaction in some very sensitive people.

With grief comes injury to the soul. I saw a lot of this in my regular clients after the events of 9/11. Many people were so profoundly shocked by what happened that day in New York, they reacted with symptoms of profound grief. These symptoms include a fear of going out of the house, insomnia, a ball sensation or tightening in the throat, or feelings of sadness and not being able to talk about it.

If the person cannot talk about anything else but this tragic event, they are in need of the sodium absorption remedy

Natrum Mur. 30th potency. If the person doesn't want to talk about it and wants everyone else to stop reminding them, they are in need of Ignatia in a 30th potency. Anyone who suffers an injury to the soul will need Arnica Montana in a single 1M potency dose.

These homeopathic remedies can relieve all of these problems and return the person to full habitation of the body, allowing a full return to sensations such as hunger, satiation, sadness and happiness.

• Math Ability

Remember Chapter 2 and the discussion of iron as a chemical needed in the brain for the ability to calculate and do math, particularly for girls? The remedy to stabolize iron in brain tissue is Ferrum Met. 1M, in one dose. Follow this with Ferrum Phos. 6X for a month or so in conjunction with a mild multiple vitamin that contains iron. This will help restore iron and stabolize this nutrient in brain tissue. Repeat this regime from time to time as needed.

With the end of fear, shame, anger and grief and the opening of the mind to the higher purposes life was meant to hold, it is possible for the individual to experience life as it was meant to be lived--with joy, understanding and inner confidence. It is at this point the concept of the ideal of the Grail becomes real.

19

Classical Homeopathy

If you have tried the remedy regime and are fascinated by the results you have achieved and want to continue to use the healing effects of remedies, you can take control of your life and take care of yourself in the little everyday things that happen to human beings by learning to use the classical system of homeopathy described in this chapter. Please do not attempt to use homeopathy in serious situations where clearly a doctor and a hospital are called for, but keeping the body in good order by reversing little problems to prevent serious problems from developing can give you a sense of control over your life and a new feeling of well being.

Also, there is no need to use homeopathy exclusively and skip doctor visits. This practice is short sighted and dangerous.

Homeopathy works very well in conjunction with conventional treatment and medicines. If your doctor finds a problem, taking the medicine prescribed and using a remedy to help the body reverse the situation can be very beneficial.

• The Classical System

The original and most often used dosing style in homeopathy is what is commonly called "Classical Homeopathy". The purpose of this system is to find the constitutional remedy of the individual. The constitution of an individual is determined to be the state of the entire person, from head to toe, as they were born into this world. This is also called the "holistic" approach to treatment because it takes a look at the entire person as a whole being, not just a particular area of the body where a problem may be occurring.

When finding an individual's constitution, it is necessary to look at signs and symptoms that cover every area of the body. One must look at the state of the mind, the pains in the head, the condition of the throat, the problems in the stomach, or bowls, or reproductive organs, and finally the extremities. All the symptoms over the entire body are analyzed. This analysis is matched to the known symptoms of a homeopathic remedy obtained through provings and listed in a Materia Medica book. When a match of an individual's symptoms is made to the symptoms a remedy can cause, that remedy is taken by the individual in a 30th potency for a period of three days. During the three-day-dosing period, the individual can expect some of their symptoms to aggravate and increase in intensity as the body works them out of the energy bodies. When all aggravations subside, the individual should experience a new state of health never before realized.

An individual comes into physical life with a set of symptoms in a constitutional pattern that deepens through life, but never really changes until the constitutional remedy is found and administered. These patterns are due to many factors which include inheritance from the genetic line, learned patterns from the family and emotional makeup through experiences in life and what we bring with us from past lives.

The constitutional remedy is the first remedy of choice for any individual. Many problems that were not known to be problems will shift after that first all-important-dose. In the example of the analogy of the orchestra from Chapter 7, the constitution can be likened to the entire orchestra playing a symphony all together at one time. If there are problems of individual musicians throughout different sections, the music will be off. The classically chosen remedy given in a single remedy dose puts everything right again. The system that is used to find the constitutional remedy of individuals can be learned by following the guidelines that follow and by practice. Remember, one cannot be harmed by taking the wrong remedy. It is just that nothing will happen.

Aggravations of existing symptoms can and do occur

and are a sign the right remedy has hit on the constitutional problem. Aggravations should last less than 24 hours and leave a person with feelings of well-being. If pain or symptoms lasts for more than 24 hours, it is not an aggravation and has nothing to do with the remedy, but rather a new problem for which the individual must seek medical attention.

• Constitutional Dosing

The single remedy system of homeopathy is the system that started with Samuel Hahnemann and was practiced by the great American homeopathic doctors of the early 20th Century. For this reason it is called the Classical System of Homeopathy. Single remedy means that only one remedy is used at a time, in the appropriate potency for the problem, according to the signs and symptoms present in the whole body. If the problem is not completely cleared and a second remedy must be chosen, the practitioner must reexamine the case and give full consideration to remedies that are listed as complements--remedies that have been determined to follow and augment the action of the first remedy--while avoiding those listed as antidotes or remedies that have been found to be detrimental to the action of the original remedy. Following this system can bring about lasting changes toward normal function and balance in the body.

The practitioner does not have to memorize millions of symptoms for hundreds of remedies. I certainly have not learned all the symptoms of every remedy. Even after 20 years of working with this system, I find that my mentor's admonition, "Never be so sure of yourself that you think you don't have to look up the symptoms. Never be prejudiced to a few remedies. Always check the books." is still the "golden rule" of homeopathy.

• Learn the Method

Any individual can learn the system and methodology of Classical Homeopathy to use for their own purposes. By using the system in conjunction with the standard homeopathic guides written by James T. Kent and William Boericke, any remedy can be found for any constitutional condition. The use of these guide books is not as complicated as it would seem by their size and complex appearance.

While other guide books to using homeopathic remedies have been written, they tend to limit their coverage to a small number of remedies to be used for a single problem. Most of these books are simply derived from classical standard guides and remedies listed for a particular symptom are printed into a smaller, more compact publication in an effort to "save time". Often, the authors of these books give the impression that years of study are necessary to use the large classical standard manuals and the smaller manuals are more appropriate for a beginner. Unfortunately, most of these compact books base their format on the disease model used by allopathic medicine. Because of this limitation, remedies suggested by these books are far too general to be matched to a specific person and often meet with limited success.

The allopathic based approach to the use of homeopathic remedies attempts to apply the allopathic medical principles in which the emphasis is placed on identifying the disease and treating the disease instead of focusing on treating the individual's symptoms. It is important to remember that the strength of classical homeopathy lies in its ability to treat all aspects of a person. Homeopathy does not and never will work as a treatment for "disease". Homeopathy is a way to treat a person that will allow that person to be restored to health and balance. With homeopathy, it is the person who must be treated--not the disease.

With the single remedy system, any symptom, no matter how strange, has a remedy for treatment and becomes a sign to the overall constitution of the individual. One does not need a diagnosis, an explanation, or an understanding of medicine to use this system. Just follow the rules, matching symptoms to remedies (forget the names of diseases) and you will find that it is possible to relieve almost any problem.

• How to Use The Materia Medica

A homeopathic Materia Medica is a book that contains a list of homeopathic remedies and the symptoms they treat. These symptoms were first caused in provings. People who were very healthy took a remedy over a period of time until the symptoms caused by the remedy appeared. This is what is known as a proving.

Homeopathic remedies are chosen for what symptoms they would cause, which is the "like cures like" principle. Due to the "like cures like" principle, homeopathic remedies are known to do the exact opposite of what they would do in the chemical form. For example, coffee is a stimulant, but a calming remedy when used as Coffea Cruda in the homeopathic form.

William Boericke wrote and published his Materia Medica in 1927. He was one of the most prominent homeopathic doctors at the time, and was also a professor of Homeopathy at the University of California. Boericke compiled provings from many sources and other Materia Medica books of his day to create a handbook that even today is the most useful Materia Medica for common use. Look for **Homeopathic Materia Medica & Repertor, by William Boericke, B.Jain Publishers, India, ISBN 81-7021-003-8.** Source information appears at the end of the chapter.

Upon opening the book, one will find the names of the remedies in bold letters and written in Latin. The use of the Latin name for the substance distinguishes the homeopathic remedy from other chemical-based forms of the same substance. The English name is underneath the Latin name in parenthesis.

The first paragraph of each entry contains a general overview of the remedy and the area of the body it works on most prominently. Many also contain information on areas that Boericke had experienced firsthand.

After this first paragraph, you will find a list of symptoms arranged in categories according to the areas of the body.

The higher parts of the body come first because they are the most important guiding symptoms. As you look at an entry in the pages--notice the list of symptoms under the 'MIND'. If there is no 'Mind' entry, the list will begin with 'HEAD'.

Most common homeopathic Materia Medica books will begin this way. The reason for this is that a remedy will begin its action on the higher parts of the body and move down to lower parts. Problems in the extremities--the legs and feet--will be listed last because they will be the last symptoms to be relieved when a remedy is taken.

If a problem is purely physical, which means it most likely stems from injury--choose a remedy that describes the physical symptoms best.

If the problem is occurring as a biochemical problem--allergies, arthritis, sleep etc.--be sure to match the mental symptoms under the 'MIND' heading to the person being treated.

This doesn't necessarily mean the mental symptoms will change unless that is the problem being treated, but in most cases--the mental makeup is the major guide to the correct remedy.

In the back of Boericke's Materia Medica is a small repertory. In the Indian Publication (the B. Jain publication printed in India) it begins on page 689.

A repertory is a list of symptoms, followed by a list of remedies that have those symptoms in its proving.

The symptom categories in the repertory also start with the mind, followed by the head, and on down the body to the extremities.

On the first page of the repertory (p. 689), the first symptom listed is **AWKWARD-Lets things fall from hand.** Remedies are listed after that in alphabetical order, and abbreviated. Since the Materia Medica is also in alphabetical order, it is not difficult to find the remedies, even if one does not understand the abbreviation.

In Boericke's Repertory, the remedies in italics are more important and have a stronger affinity to the symptoms than remedies in regular type.

On page 689, under **AWKWARD**--*Apis, Bov,* and *Nat.M* are in italics. If you wanted to find the remedy that most matched your awkward person, you would go to each of these remedies in the Materia Medica until you were satisfied with one remedy that matched most of characteristics of the person.

Go to the Materia Medica section of the book and turn to 'Apis' on page 61. The first sentence in that entry tells you where the remedy has the most influence. Read through the symptoms of the remedy. Don't be inhibited by medical terminology. Most entries are common sense and easy to read. The entries in italics are more important than regular type sentences. If you can find 5 to 6 sentences throughout the list of symptoms that match the symptoms of the person who is sick, it is well indicated for them. The person doesn't have to display all the symptoms in the list, just one, and 5 to 6 other symptom from the overall entry for a particular remedy.

For example, if a person matches the
"awkward; drops things readily" symptom in the '**MIND'**
the "vertigo worse when closing the eyes" in the '**HEAD'**
the "stinging pains" in the '**THROAT'**
the "extremely tender" symptoms in the '**ABDOMEN'**
and "hoarseness" in the '**RESPIRATORY'** it would be a well indicated remedy and should relieve not only these problems but many more which were not necessarily thought of as problems. If one can find other symptoms that match, the remedy is even more indicated.

• Practice

The more one practices looking up symptoms in the repertory and reading remedies in the Materia Medica, the more familiar one can get with remedies and matching them to people.

Start with any symptom in any part of the body, but it should be the most prominent physical symptom--the one giving the most pain or the biggest problem at this time.

It seems to work best to choose a physical symptom to look up first rather than a mental symptom because physical symptoms are typically more distinctive.

Next, find the symptom in the repertory, look at the list of remedies and find the italicized ones. Next, turn to the Materia Medica section of the book and study each remedy, until you find the one that matches more symptoms over all. You can't miss finding the remedy that will be most helpful when you use this method.

Be sure to match a mental symptom in the Mind section to the person being repertorized. It may not be what you start with when you look up symptoms in the repertory, but it is still the most important guiding symptom. The rate of success will be much higher if this is remembered.

• Kent's Repertory

The Repertory of the Homeopathic Materia Medica, (B. Jain Publishers of India, ISBN 81-7021-059-3) written by Dr. James T. Kent can be used in the same way to complement the Materia Medica. Kent's Repertory is a huge work, covering many, many symptoms. If you are fascinated by homeopathy and wish to continue to study, you will find Kent's Repertory very interesting.

To use the repertory, look up the symptoms one by one by heading starting with the higher parts of the body and moving to lower areas. In other words, the symptom of a headache is more important than the symptom of foot pain, unless the foot pain in the most prominent symptom.

As you find a particular pain symptom with a characteristic quality, such a 'pain in the forehead that throbs' you will see a list of all the remedies that describe that type of pain. As you go further in the column, you will see more and more specific situations where that pain may occur. This gives you many possible and idiosyncratic symptoms in order to match the best situation to the person suffering the pain. The remedies written in bold print are the most often used remedies for that symptom, italicized remedies are the next most common, and the remedies written in plain print are the least often used. However, if you find a very specific situation, such as 'pain in the forehead that throbs when lying in the dark' and there is only one remedy listed, and that remedy is written in plain print, that remedy will still be a perfect remedy match to the constitution of the person who experiences that pain. Looking up the remedy in the Materia Medica will confirm that there are symptoms related to that person in many headings of that specific remedy.

• New Symptoms

After the remedy you have chosen is taken, the symptoms may be relieved, but it is also possible for a new symptom to become prominent. When this happens, more than one remedy is required for complete relief. Look up the new symptoms in the repertory. Look at the remedies listed under it, and find a match to the new problems, again matching the mental symptom as well.

• Relationships

In the back of Boericke's Materia Medica starting on page 1080 (the B. Jain publication only) there is a chart called "**The Relationship of Remedies with Duration of Action**". Look up the remedy you took first in the left hand column. Next, look to see if there is a relationship to the remedy you plan to take next. If the new remedy is found in the column labeled "Complements" or "Remedies that Follow Well", you can expect good results because the second remedy helps to continue and promote the reaction begun by the first. "Inimicals" are remedies that do not follow each other well and will give an adverse reaction. Be certain that you do **not** use an inimical after your first remedy. Antidotes can also be compatibles, but taking an antidote to the first remedy will stop any further beneficial action. If two remedies have no relationship, there is no problem in taking one after the other.

• Be Patient

The column that has the "**Duration**" of action of the remedy is very important. Each remedy has duration of action. That means that if you take one dose or several, the reaction will continue in your body for the number of days listed in the column. This does not mean that you take it for the number of days listed. It means that you must consider when taking a remedy that it will continue working for only one day or sixty days depending. Anything you take after the first remedy should be compatible. If it is not, the curative action may be interrupted. It also means that one should be patient and let the remedies work.

Many times the best action takes place up to a week after you have taken a remedy. It is difficult at times, but we must resist the temptation to take more and more remedies because that is the way we have learned from taking conventional medicine. With homeopathy, the effect is just the opposite. One takes only a little, and the action can continue for a long time afterwards. The problem doesn't return when you stop taking the remedy as it can with herbs or conventional medicine.

• How to Take Remedies

In general, if you take a 12th potency, take it three times a day for a week. If you take a 30th potency, take it three times a day for three days. If you take a 200th potency--take only one dose. If it is a 1M or 1000 potency, take only one dose in a month. Most often, the constitutional remedy is taken in a 30th potency for three days only.

After the doses are taken, let them act--and you will notice things come and go, and then subside completely as the remedy works its curative action. If an uncomfortable aggravation occurs, take an extra dose to help the body work through the problem. This is much more effective than backing off as one would in allopathic treatment. Remember, there is no drug side effect, just an energy impulse clearing the problem.

To take a homeopathic remedy, place 4 or 5 of the little pellets under the tongue and let them dissolve. Do not have anything in the mouth fifteen minutes before and after taking the remedy. Do not swallow the pellets with water or anything else-- just place them dry under the tongue and let them dissolve.

• Caution in Repeating Remedies

If the symptoms have gone away, but return later in a changed form, you may repeat the same remedy taken earlier, but there must be caution. If you repeat the same remedy while its duration of action is still working, you can antidote the effect and it will be very difficult to get a good reaction started again. The best thing to do is to take a complement before repeating the remedy--so the actions of the two doses of the same remedy don't clash. The other and more preferable course of action is to move to the next higher potency.

That is--if you took ARSENICUM ALBUM 30C for an allergy problem, and the allergy went away for a while, but returned after two weeks in a lesser or slightly different form, one would not repeat ARSENICUM 30C right away. The action of ARSENICUM can go on acting for 60 to 90 days--and there is no way to know how long it is acting in each individual. The first dose can bring up multiple small aggravations while it is hitting old problems embedded in energy bodies. Repeating the same potency while the first dose is still acting will cause the energy of those doses to smash into each other, ending the action of both and making it very difficult to get that remedy to work in that individual again. If you must repeat a remedy, take a complement--such as APIS or BELLADONNA in the case of ARSENICUM for example--to offset the action of the first dose.

If the symptoms for which you first took ARSENICUM never return, do not repeat it for several months at least, and only if new symptoms lead you to choose it for a different problem. Once a remedy has worked to relieve problems, repeating it while it is still working will bring back the problems--perhaps permanently. So--if you are tempted to help the remedy along a little--since it did so well to help the problem in the first place--**don't.**

• The Potency is Too High

If ARSENICUM 30 worked beautifully for a short period of time but the symptoms returned exactly as they were in the beginning, it may be that the 30 was too high a potency to get to the energy body that was affected. You can't go to a lower potency straight away, since you would get the drainage effect of a chord potency. You could use a complement first, then drop to a lower potency of ARSENICUM such as a 12 after the complement, and see if that helps relieve the symptoms on a more permanent basis. Since ARSENICUM ALBUM is a poison, it is not commonly available nor is it advisable to take it in a potency lower than a 9C.

• What About Antidotes

Many people have read or been told by other people who use homeopathy that strong smelling substances will antidote remedies. Many people avoid trying homeopathic remedies because the restrictions and diet they have been told they must follow while under homeopathic care seems so austere. In actual fact, homeopathic remedies are energetic and do not interact on the physical realm.

There is a chart on Page 1080 of the B.Jain publication of Boericke's Materia Medica (The Gibson Miller Chart) that gives the duration of action of each remedy along with a list of antidotes. Some remedies list COFF. as an antidote. Where this is listed, the remedy could be antidoted by COFFEA CRUDA as a homeopathic remedy, but not by coffee as the gross material substance you drink in the morning.

Homeopathic remedies should not be exposed to excessive heat (temperatures over 150 degrees F.), cold (below freezing), or contaminated by food items (such as juice being spilled on them). Nor should they be placed in containers that have been previously used for another purpose. Beyond these cautions, there is nothing that will affect the action of a homeopathic remedy after it is taken.

When a remedy is working, nothing material will antidote it. I have never known a well chosen remedy to be easily antidoted by normal life activities. Caffeine has never presented a problem in my experience. Using mint toothpaste has not created a problem as long as it was not used within half an hour of taking the remedy.

Some homeopathic practitioners have blamed common substances for antidoting remedies as a way to explain why a remedy didn't work. These homeopathic practitioners are probably in the habit of using very high potencies for physical problems. If the potency is too high, it skirts by the energy body affected giving a temporary amelioration of symptoms, but symptoms will return only because the potency was too high, not because it was antidoted by a material substance.

• Where to Buy Remedies and Books

On the internet: Many web sites sell remedies.

In Southern California:

Clark's Nutrition Center in Riverside at (951) 686-4757, in San Bernardino at (909) 885-7165 and Loma Linda (909) 478-7714.

Any remedy can be mail ordered from Capitol Drugs and sent anywhere in the country. Call them at 1-800-858-8833. Visit Capitol Drugs in West Hollywood on Santa Monica Blvd.

Wellspring Books in Claremont carries some remedies.

Sprout's in Temecula also has many remedies.

B.J.'s in the High Desert communities has 6X potency remedies and will order more.

There are health food stores throughout San Bernardino, Riverside, Los Angeles and Orange Counties that carry remedies. Look in your local Yellow Pages.

• From the manufacturer:

If you want to go directly to the manufacturer, start with The Standard Homeopathic Co. This is a very old and very well established manufacturer in the L.A. area. They are the makers of the Hyland Cell Salt remedies which are most of the 6X potencies you will need. Call Standard at 1-800-624-9659.

Another manufacturer where you can order directly is the Boiron Company. This is an old French company that now has a plant in California. Call Boiron at 1-800-258-8823.

Another very good company is Dolisos in Las Vegas. This is also an older French company that now makes products in the U.S. From Dolisos, you can purchase all of the other higher potency remedies if you could not get them from other sources. Call 1-800-DOLISOS.

- Books

The homeopathic practitioner books can be ordered from The Standard Company or Dolisos as mentioned above. Many web sites exist where one can find these and many other homeopathic books.

- On the Web

If you wish to do more research on homeopathy, there are many web sites dedicated to the subject and the experiences of individuals using the remedies. There are also many sites that sell remedies and books.

Be forewarned, the internet can be a very confusing place. While there is much information available in the area of alternative and complementary health, opinions and advice may not always reflect what is good for the body. Before making any decisions about trying an alternative health care regime, just think how your body will react and try to choose the system that seems the most gentle with the advice that will set things right and not further aggrivate already existing problems.

20

Acute Dosing For Common Problems

L ook again at the model of the orchestra you have already read in Chapter 7. Classical homeopathy and the constitution of the individual is likened to an entire orchestra participating in the production of a symphony that is the blended sound of each member of the orchestra. Every individual person can identify a constitutional remedy that will describe their physical characteristics perfectly. The use of that one constitutional remedy will clear many problems and restore many missing energy patterns, allowing the person to live life in harmony such as the sound produced by an orchestra whose members are playing to the best of their ability.

The drums in a piece of music are another example. Every orchestra, every band, every traditional form of music that exists utilizes the sound of drums. Drums are instruments that are universal to every form of music. In the same sense, there are homeopathic remedies that are universal and work the same for every individual who takes them, no matter the state of the person's health or the pattern of their constitution. These universal remedies can be taken in doses of short duration to stop acute illness or to lessen the effect of injury. Many people in the entertainment industry use these remedies to keep going.

• Universal Remedy Solutions

• Cold and Flu

At the time one may begin to feel the effects of a cold or the flu virus, when the throat is just beginning the feel scratchy or sore, when the body may be just beginning to feel achy, or a fever is just beginning to bring on a headache, it is possible to throw the flu or cold virus out of the energy bodies my using a product call **Oscillococcinum®** made by the Boiron Company. This product is sold in a white box with orange bands on the front. Inside the box are little tubes filled with tiny pellets. Taking a dose of about one fourth of the tube, three times in a 12 hour period can throw the virus out the energy bodies by targeting the immune system to fight the invading virus before it gets a hold on the physical body. If it does not work to completely eliminate the virus, it will help to lessen the effect and shorten the duration of the illness. Sometimes it happens that the immune system of an individual does not recognize a virus at all and has no defense against it. This is the situation where an illness will develop in spite of everything used to stop it.

If one continues to develop the illness after using Oscillococcinum®, one may still have a chance to throw off the virus by using **Aconitum Nap**. in a 200 potency. Take this remedy three times in one hour--that is once on the hour, once at the half-hour, and again on the hour. This acute dosing style is very effective in most cases to stop a flu virus in its tracks. If one only has a 30th potency on hand, the same effect may be achieved by taking a dose of the 30th potency every 10 minutes for an hour or two. Stop taking it when you begin to feel better. Also, **Zincum Met**. in a 6X will help boost the immune system to help throw off the illness. Use Zincum Met. 6X after the one hour acute dosing for Aconitum Nap. is complete.

On the rare occasions when these three remedies have not stopped the flu or cold from developing because the immune system did not recognize any part of the invading virus, it is possible to shorten the duration of the illness by alternating doses of Natrum Mur. with Arsencum Album. Keep a 30th potency of each of these remedies on hand for this purpose. Take them in alternating doses every 10 minutes for an hour, and every few hours for the next 24 hours.

It is also possible to treat symptoms with other individual remedies after this 24 hour period if the illness is still lingering on. Kali Bichromium is useful for a stuffy runny nose. Pulsatilla is good if the nose is just runny. Antimonium Crude is very helpful if there is chest congestion. However, do not hesitate to see a doctor is symptoms are severe.

Oscillococcinum® may be taken once a month as a preventative to viral infection, however, repeating it within the month after it is taken can antidote the effect. Mark your calendar at the time you take it. If you have taken Oscillococcinum® within that month and flu-like symptoms develop, **do not repeat it.** Instead, go on to the other remedies for boosting your immune system against the flu. Zincum Met. 6X would be a good choice and Aconitum Nap. 200 if symptoms continue to develop.

• Sudden Injury

Because there is always the possibility of sudden unexpected injury, it is wise to keep Arnica Montana on hand. In the case of injury, Arnica Montana in a 30th potency, taken every 10 minutes for up to 2 hours as soon as possible after an injury can lessen the severity and speed healing. If a 200th potency is available, take it every 10 minutes for one hour.

This style of dosing works to lessen the impact of the injury because injury causes damage over time as the impact penetrates through the energy bodies from the outside toward the internal. Before the full extent of the injury has penetrated all levels of the energy bodies, it is possible to throw the effect off of the outer most energy bodies and modify severity.

If the injury is severe enough to require stitches, surgery or casting, do not expect Arnica to offset the need for treatment or lull a person into believing they do not need to see a doctor. Homeopathy cannot completely reverse that sort of damage to the physical body. Arnica can offset the effect of bruising, relieve much of the pain, or stop swelling before it develops. However, seek medical aid as soon as possible when it is need. The use of Arnica will speed healing and shorten recovery after the medical procedure.

If there is head injury, alternate Arnica Montana with any potency of Natrum Sulph. This remedy helps prevent swelling which can lead to concussion after head trauma.

Surgery--**Arnica Montana 6X potency or the 30th potency--**The use of this remedy increases the body's ability to heal and handle the changes the body endures in surgery. When using Arnica Montana, recovery time is remarkable fast. Most commonly, this remedy used before surgery is taken in doses of 2 pellets at a time in a 30th (either x or c) potency 3 times a day. Begin two days before surgery and continue for five days after.

For the healing of wounds on the surface of the skin such as incisions, cuts and scrapes, use **Calendula** in the gel, cream and ointment forms.

Pain--Homeopathic remedies do not have influence over the body as drugs do. They cannot block or overshadow pain, but one remedy, **Hypericum Perf.,** can help calm nerve endings to relieve some pain. Hypericum is usually taken 2 pellets at a time in a 30th (either x or c) potency 3 times a day for 3 days.

Hypericum is also a good remedy to help heal damaged nerves, alternate with **Salicylicum Acidum,** also in a 30th potency, at different times of the day.

• Burns

Because the pure substance known as **Cantharis** can cause burns on the skin, in a homeopathic potency Cantharis can help relieve the effects of a burn. Taken in a 30th potency, every 10 minutes for an hour, this remedy can actually lesson the severity of burns and cause the area of the skin affected to begin immediate healing. A first degree burn could disappear entirely with no redness or pain after a few doses. A second degree burn could be prevented from blistering and pain decreased after several doses. A third degree burn will require treatment from a doctor, but the Cantharis will lesson severity a great deal and allow for quick healing.

Cantharis can also be very helpful in the case of sunburn since this can occur over a large area of the skin. The best results will be achieved when the remedy is taken as soon as possible after exposure. It is also possible to take a few preventive doses before spending a long period of time in the sun in order to prevent burning. It this case, one can take a 30th potency dose once every few hours during the day, increasing to short frequent doses as the time of exposure increases. If the person begins to feel dizzy, this can be the proving effect of Cantharis and doses should be stopped all together.

• Eating Disorders

Not eating--A person who is not eating as from an eating disorder, grief, or after surgery, **Zincum Metallicum** in a 30th potency, usually one or two doses is all that is needed to restore the appetite. In overload from too much supplementation, Zinc can cause an increase in appetite as the body attempts to dilute the overload. Stop Zinc supplementation and use Zincum Met. 30th three times a day for three days.

If there is the symptom of nausea, or one suspects a mild food poisoning, or needs to antidote or detox the effects of a drug, or to detox the drugs used as anesthetic, **Nux Vomica** is the remedy. This is taken in a 2 pellet dose, 30th potency, three times a day for 3 days.

For morning Sickness---**Carbo Veg. 6X or 6C,** helps to settle the stomach. Take a 2 pellet dose as needed.

Motion Sickness---**Cocculus 6X or 6C,** take a 2 pellet dose any time and as often as needed before and during the journey.

• West Nile Virus

The West Nile Virus is a new concern in the Continental United States. Southern California experienced a serious outbreak in the summer of 2004 where 714 cases were reported with 19 deaths. Further spread of the virus is expected in the future.

The West Nile Virus is transmitted to humans in the bite of infected mosquitoes. Authorities say that the majority of people bitten by infected mosquitoes will not develop any type of illness. It is estimated that about 20% of the people bitten will develop the symptoms of the disease. These symptoms include headache, high fever, neck stiffness, weakness and disorientation. In very few cases, the infection progresses to encephalitis or meningitis. However, those who have reported being ill with the disease have reported a lengthier and more debilitating illness than anticipated with symptoms lasting up to 30 days and recover taking as much as two months. Since this disease is likely to continue to be a problem and efforts at mosquito control are usually only partially successful, boosting immunity to protect the individual from developing the illness even if bitten is a good idea.

Since West Nile Virus infects birds before it is passed to humans and other mammals through the bite of the mosquito, it makes sense that **Oscillococcinum®** could be used to boost personal immunity to ward of this illness in people whose immune system is normal and functions correctly. Oscillococcinum® is a remedy homeopathically potentized from the immune carrying internal organs of a duck. Since viruses commonly incubate in fowl, this immune enhancing characteristic of fowl can be passed to humans who use this remedy. As stated earlier, Oscillococcinum® is made by the Boiron Company and is commonly available in health food stores, vitamin pharmacies and many grocery stores. For protection against West Nile Virus during the summer months when infection is most likely, an individual may take a dose of 10 to 12 pellets, under the tongue three times in 12 hours, once a month. Since this is a 200th potency, it will not be effective in children less than 2 years of age--since the energy body relating to the 200th potency does not develop until age two. Also, since this product is the product made from a duck, a person who may be allergic to chicken, duck, goose or other fowl products, should avoid this remedy.

If the symptoms of West Nile Virus do develop, do not hesitate to see a doctor for treatment. Many advances in treating this illness have been developed recently. **Do not take Oscillococcinum® more often than once a month.** Mark your calendar when you take it and do not repeat it within the month even if symptoms do develop.

• Menopausal problems

A few years ago the results of studies made on hormone replacement therapy for menopausal women were released to the public. Many women felt confused as to whether hormones would be available to them during the onset of menopausal symptoms or whether they would have to suffer without since the use of hormones was found to increase the risk of heart disease and stroke. This was very confusing since the therapy had been recommended to reduce the risk of these two medical problems. Many women who did not intent to take replacement hormones were talked into it with the promise they would be protected from future heart and blood vessel problems, leaving many dazed and disillusioned and still suffering with symptoms.

It is my experience that most women who have problems during menopause usually find relief with the homeopathic remedy **Sulphur**. Sulfur as a necessary nutrient which is responsible for the proper viscosity of body fluids. Being deficient in sulfur in the cells of the body leads to night sweats, late-night sleeplessness, recurring sinus infections—all the usual symptoms associated with the menopausal time of life. To relieve these annoying symptoms, Sulphur 30, taken three times a day for three days along with the nutritional supplement MSM (purchased in capsules of 1000mgs) helps body cells absorb sulfur properly, thereby eliminating annoying symptoms.

Using the calcium and magnesium remedies in the regime described in Chapter 16 also helps to eliminate the other symptoms associated with menopause, such as osteoporosis, blood vessel integrity problems, heart disease associated symptoms--as well as migraine headaches due to hormonal inbalance that can occur or recur at menopause.

Bibliography

This is a list of books used as a reference source in the writing of this book.

Boericke, William, M.D., <u>Homeopathic Materia Medica and Repertory</u>, B. Jain Publishers, New Delhi,India, Reprint Edition 1995

Handley, Rima, <u>A Homeopathic Love Story,</u> North Atlantic Books, Berkeley, CA1990

Kent, J.T., <u>Repertory of the Homoeopathic Materia Medica</u>, B. Jain Publishers, New Delhi, India, Reprint Edition 1995

Hahnemann, Samuel, <u>The Organon of Medicine</u>, translated by William Boericke, M.D. B. Jain Publishers, New Delhi, India

Qureshi, Masood, <u>Principles of Homeopathy for Medical Students,</u> Masood Publications, Lahore, Pakistan 1980

The methodology explained in this book does not necessarily reflect the methods used by other homeopathic practitioners, schools and communities, but rather is the method developed by Michele Iqbal exclusively through experience and experimentation over a period of more than twenty years. This is not to say other works on the subject of homeopathy are not worth reading. On the contrary, many books focus on problems and how to solve them, which can be very valuable to anyone who wishes to use homeopathy to prevent future illness. However, there are some methods written in other works on homeopathy which the reader must understand will not work correctly if used and should be avoided. These methods include using potencies of 1M or 10M for constitutional (chronic) problems, using combinations for chronic problems and using any remedy labeled homeopathic that is taken in any way other than under the tongue such as injection or capsules to be swallowed into the stomach, unless the capsule contains the liquid tincture of a remedy known to work in a 1X potency,

I do not provide a list of other homeopathic books simply because there are too many to choose from and many new ones that are published all the time. Do not hesitate to explore the library, Internet or local bookstore for further reading on the subject.

About The Author

Michele Iqbal grew up in the State of Washington where her father practiced veterinary medicine in the city of Seattle. She is a graduate of the University of California at Davis with a degree in Fine Arts.

Dr. Iqbal was living in Pakistan in the 1980's with her Pakistani born husband and three children when she discovered the wonderful healing qualities of homeopathy. Her first homeopathic doctor, Dr. Abdul Rehman, was able to cure her son of autism. She apprenticed with this extraordinary individual and learned a great deal about the true nature of the effect of homeopathy on the human body.

Dr. Iqbal went on to complete a Ph.D. degree, a Diploma of Homeopathic Medical Sciences (D.H.M.S.) from the National College of Homeopathy in Rawalpindi, Pakistan, and is licensed by the Government of Pakistan as a Homeopathic Practitioner.

In addition, Michele Iqbal holds a California Teaching Credential, has taught in the L.A. Unified School District and the Fontana Unified School District. She has taught Homeopathy for Curentur University in Santa Monica, worked for Capital Drugs in West Hollywood as an advice practitioner, and has practiced privately in Riverside, California.

Dr. Iqbal is no longer in private homeopathic practice, but rather plans to concentrate on publishing and bringing her knowledge and experience to a worldwide audience.

Dr. Iqbal plans to write many more works of practical homeopathic advice. These books will soon be available on her website, micheleiqbal.com and through totalwellnesspublishing. com.

Michele has recently published **Jake: A Soul's Journey Through Time**, a book of inspiration in dealing with the loss of a loved one by the realization that souls very often stay with us through many lifetimes.

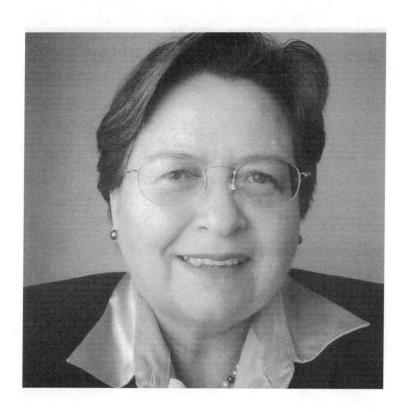

Also by Dr. Iqbal:

Jake: A Soul's Journey Through Time

An inspirational story of losing a loved on and knowing they are still with us